Transforming Presence

The Difference That Nursing Makes

Transforming Presence

The Difference That Nursing Makes

By

Margaret A. Newman,
RN, PhD, FAAN

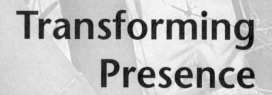

F. A. DAVIS COMPANY • Philadelphia

F. A. Davis Company
1915 Arch Street
Philadelphia, PA 19103
www.fadavis.com

Printed in the United States of America

Last digit indicates print number: 10 9 8 7 6 5 4 3 2 1

Publisher: Joanne Patzek DaCunha, RN, MSN
Project Editor: Kristin L. Kern
Art and Design Manager: Carolyn O'Brien

As new scientific information becomes available through basic and clinical research, recommended treatments and drug therapies undergo changes. The author(s) and publisher have done everything possible to make this book accurate, up to date, and in accord with accepted standards at the time of publication. The author(s), editors, and publisher are not responsible for errors or omissions or for consequences from application of the book, and make no warranty, expressed or implied, in regard to the contents of the book. Any practice described in this book should be applied by the reader in accordance with professional standards of care used in regard to the unique circumstances that may apply in each situation. The reader is advised always to check product information (package inserts) for changes and new information regarding dose and contraindications before administering any drug. Caution is especially urged when using new or infrequently ordered drugs.

Library of Congress Cataloging-in-Publication Data
Newman, Margaret A.
 Transforming presence : the difference that nursing makes / by
Margaret A. Newman.
       p. ; cm.
 Includes bibliographical references and index.
 ISBN-13: 978-0-8036-1752-0
 ISBN-10: 0-8036-1752-6
 1. Nursing—Philosophy. 2. Health—Philosophy. I. Title.
 [DNLM: 1. Holistic Nursing. 2. Health Care Reform. WY 86.5 N554t 2008]
 RT84.5.N483 2008
 610.73–dc22   2007030695

Acknowledgment

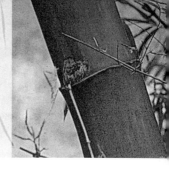

I am truly grateful for colleagues who gave of their time and expertise to review the manuscript of this book. They are: Dr. Emiko Endo, Dr. Dorothy Jones, Dr. Margaret Dexheimer Pharris, Dr. Marlaine Smith, Dr. Cheryl Stegbauer, and Dr. Janet Williamson. They helped me to stay on track and provided valuable input to the comprehensiveness of the work.

M.A.N.

Reviewers

Jacqueline Fawcett, RN, PhD, FAAN
Professor
University of Massachusetts
Boston, Massachusetts

Kristen Montgomery, RN, PhD
Former Professor
University of South Carolina

Marilyn E. Parker, RN, PhD, FAAN
Professor
Florida Atlantic University
Boca Raton, Florida

Mary Elizabeth Sadler, RN, PhD
Professor
Indiana University of Pennsylvania
Indiana, Pennsylvania

Patricia Schaefer, RN, PhD
Associate Professor
Grand Valley State University
Grand Rapids, Michigan

Figures

Contents

Introduction

The forces of the field of energy . . . interoscillate through the symmetry of equilibrium to various asymmetries, never pausing at equilibrium.

Buckminster Fuller, 1975

I find myself feeling uncertain about the next steps in the development of the theory of health as expanding consciousness (Newman, 1979; 1986; 1994), but at the same time wanting to move on. I recognize this feeling as an aspect of transition into the unknown. As one begins to experience the transformation of moving away from an old familiar stage of development to a new unfamiliar stage, the doubts and uncertainties arise. The old rules don't work anymore. One thinks it would be easier, safer to revert to the former way of doing and seeing things and avoid the pain and discomfort of uncertainty. But that is no longer possible. New possibilities have arisen and one must move on. There was no turning back from Copernicus' view of the solar system. There is no turning back from the perspective of health as expanding consciousness. I am encouraged by Skolimowski (1994), who experienced the process of unfolding knowledge as traumatic and reminded us that only the guardians of the status quo remain confident, in their refusal to recognize new insights.

Asymmetry[1] in art and design is very appealing to me. A while back I explored its relevance in other fields and found that asymmetry may be coded in the human organism at its most elementary stage. Geschwind and Galaburda (1985), experts in the field of cerebral lateralization, described a number of examples of asymmetry in nature. For instance, the

---

[1] Symmetry refers to a similarity of form on each side of a midline; asymmetry connotes a difference of form (or function) from side to side.

lobster, early in life, has two symmetrical small claws, called pincers. One of the pincers enlarges and becomes a crusher. The mechanism of transformation from pincer to crusher is a chance event: the availability of something to crush. If one of the pincers has the opportunity to crush an oyster shell, it becomes the crusher. Information from the pincer that crushes initiates a process of suppressing the transformative potential of the opposite pincer. Being a pincer or becoming a crusher? There are similar transforming points in each of our lives. Opportunities for choice occur for each of us, and in our unique way we respond. This action differentiates us from another person exposed to seemingly similar circumstances.

Asymmetry has something to do with development, with moving on. Emerson (1860, p. 192 Beauty), like Fuller (previously quoted), spoke to the notion of disturbing the equilibrium:

> Beautiful as is the symmetry of any form, if the form can move, we seek a more excellent symmetry. The interruption of equilibrium stimulates the eye to desire restoration of asymmetry. . . . This is the theory of dancing, to recover continually in changes the lost equilibrium, not by abrupt and angular, but by gradual and curving movements.

The process is one of going from asymmetry to asymmetry, or instability to instability. The process is one of peaks and troughs, order and disorder, unfolding at higher levels.

If we follow the oft-touted advice to strive for balance in all things—a steady state, equilibrium, we may miss the opportunity for growth that disruption offers. Prigogine, Nobel laureate, said that "at equilibrium, matter is blind. . . . Far from equilibrium, it may begin to see" (Brain/Mind Bulletin, 1986). He pointed out that DNA molecules are evidence of "broken symmetry" since they can be read in only one direction, like a human language. In other words, instability creates purposeful activity and direction. We come to a point at which the old rules don't work anymore, and we must make a choice. There is no turning back to the safety and comfort of our old ways of doing things. The asymmetry of expanding consciousness is important to our understanding of the life process and health. It is an asymmetrical choice to move on.

In nursing, the emphasis is on relationship: relationships within the client's life and relationship between the nurse and the client. A relationship may be symmetrical, complementary, or asymmetrical. A symmetrical relationship is one in which the action of one party escalates the action of the other, as in competition. Complementary relationships tend to move toward equilibrium: the action of one balances the action of another, as in dominance-submission (Bateson, 1972). An asymmetrical relationship is one of growth, evolvement, and transcendence. Movement of a symmetrical or complementary relationship to an asymmetrical one requires additional information and new insight, an expansion of consciousness. For instance, a young woman, when relating her story of divorce from her first husband, viewed it as a failure in her life, but subsequently when helped to take a look at the trajectory of her life pattern, she saw how that event opened new opportunities for her and began to regard it as a stepping stone, a turning point. The insight of additional information made the difference.

This is a book about a theory of health: a theory that emerged from a nursing perspective and is transforming nursing practice. Martha Rogers' revolutionary writings in the 1960s resonated with my own experience of nursing and prompted me to pursue graduate study with her. Once in dialogue with Martha, I was challenged by her insistence that health and illness were *simply* expressions of the life process, one no more important than the other. For one submerged in a disease-oriented health model, that concept was difficult to grasp. Martha's assertion compelled me to think beyond the then current concepts of health.

About that time I gained insight from the experience of a friend who had been diagnosed with hyperthyroidism, was not responding to medical treatment, and was facing the possibility of surgery. Before pursuing that alternative, she was seen by Dora Kunz (1991), a person who could visualize the flow of energy of a person's interactions (Weber, 1984). Dora could see that my friend's energy was being diffused in every direction and concluded that it was not relevant to tell her to curtail her activities to conserve or channel her energy because this pattern represented her way of life. Dora did suggest that my friend make sure she took in enough energy to sustain this pattern. It was true that my friend expended her energy in many directions: in favors to friends and colleagues, in an overcommitment to her work, and in response to the needs of a large family. She often skipped meals and got little rest because of her packed schedule. When I really began to think about it, her thyroid gland was trying to keep up with her demands. The medical/surgical approach to diminish or delete the activity of the gland ran counter to what she was trying to accomplish. Dora's vision was to work with the pattern rather than against it.

Subsequently my friend was able to heed Dora's advice, did not need the surgery, and was able to greatly reduce her medications. The transforming factor, I submit, was the *insight* she gained regarding her own pattern. The pattern that eventually manifested itself as disease was *primary*. Her disease was a manifestation of the whole, not a separate entity to be attacked as though it were alien to the person. It revealed information about the person-environment relationships, and was meaningful in my friend's evolving consciousness.

A new concept of health was emerging: a unitary (indivisible) process of expanding consciousness, moving through various configurations, including disease and disruption. Martha Rogers, for a while, considered this view particulate, but shortly before her death acknowledged consciousness as the pattern of the whole (Rogers, 1995). I never had any doubts.

In the early development of the theory, the research was limited by the constraints of the scientific method. My colleagues and I pointedly tried to select concepts considered parameters of wholeness (Newman, 1979), like movement and time perception, but forced them into fixed operational definitions and controlled circumstances. We were still trying to force round pegs into square holes: unitary concepts into reductionist methods. The results yielded little understanding of the *experience* of persons in situations of altered movement (Newman, 1972). Fortunately in the debriefing interviews characteristic of an experiment of this type, the participants shared their experience of consciously compensating for the effect of movement on time perception, and I began to move away from the supposed control and objectivity I thought so important at the time.

Rogers' (1970) emphasis on *mutual process* signaled emphasis on the relational process as the phenomenon of inquiry, a focus that required a change in the way we do research. But old habits die hard. It took a while for us to move from an observer-observed focus on the client to the mutuality of the nurse-client relationship in research as well as in practice. As the transformative nature of nursing practice asserted itself, the focus had to be revised to depict the *process* of the evolving pattern of the whole (Newman, 1997). Anecdotal evidence from married women in a semirural setting (Newman, 1986) revealed the concepts of movement, time, space, and consciousness as dimensions of meaningful relationships. These women, whose interaction with others was characterized by submission, resentment, and distancing, had little or no *movement* outside their homes except for work and little or no *space* or *time* for themselves. The notion of *pattern of the whole* emerged as the important focus of health (Newman, 1983; 1986).

Recognizing the open-ended, dynamic nature of reality, I was motivated to do participatory research. As I plunged in, I was amazed to discover meaningful directions emerging from the deluge of data regarding the transformation of both the researched and the researcher in relation to practice. The assumptions of disease as a manifestation of pattern, pattern as a manifestation of evolving consciousness, and mutuality of the process, guided the quest for a way to examine the theory of health as expanding consciousness. Throughout the process of pattern recognition, the focus was on meaning; that is, meaningfulness of the pattern to the client. We had to give up predictability as an outcome of research. Prigogine's (1976) theory of dissipative structures was helpful in seeing that we cannot know in advance which direction the process will take. The answer lies in staying present in the process until understanding and transformation of the experience for both client/participant and nursing practitioner/researcher occurs. This takes courage and an awareness in the moment. The greater relevance is in the universality of the experience rather than the generality of it. The difference between these points is discussed in Chapter 4.

Having given up control and predictability, and being entered fully into the relationship of mutual process, I realized that what we were doing as research was the process of practice and acknowledged the role of theory a priori (Newman, 1990). It was praxis—the merging of theory, research, and practice. Similarities with other established methods can be seen (e.g., participatory, hermeneutic, dialectic, heuristic) but the praxis of HEC is not confined to any of these. It emerges from the nature of the theory and is transforming for all involved.

A physician once said to me, "What you're talking about would revolutionize medical care." At the time, I thought, I'd be satisfied with a revolution of nursing care. And, apparently, that is what is occurring: Capasso (2005), after experiencing the transformative power of the theory in practice, echoed that "... the adoption of a Newman model would revolutionize nursing practice."

We are the revolution! I trust that the experiences and research upon which this book is based will be meaningful to you and when incorporated in your practice, will make a difference in your life.

Chapter 1

A New Concept of Health

The concept of health as the absence of disease is an admirable, but often unobtainable goal. Even programs of health promotion, or disease prevention, do not fulfill this goal. Persons who follow all the rules still find themselves suddenly disrupted by heart attack, stroke, unexplained cancer, or other debilitating diseases. We need a new concept of health.

The seed of the idea of a unitary concept of health was sown during my experience as the primary caregiver for my mother, who had amyotrophic lateral sclerosis.[1] My mother, a previously active businesswoman with multiple ties to community organizations, searched in vain for a cure. Eventually it became painfully clear that she and our family just had to learn to live with her losses. My experience was one of learning to live day by day. There was no past or future. I became aware of my mother's presence as a whole person, not someone defined by her disabilities. As a 20-year-old recent college graduate, I was looking forward to developing a career and moving out in the world, but I found my life circumscribed by my relationship to my mother. Her movement in space and time was restricted. My movement in space and time was restricted. I came to know her in a deep and meaningful way.

At the time of her death 5 years later, I was aware that the direction of my life was changing. It was a turning point and a choice point. I thought I could resume my previous ways of living for myself and my own striving as a young adult, but I was confronted with a new path,

---

[1]A degenerative disease of the motor neurons, better known as Lou Gehrig's disease. Also portrayed vividly in *Tuesdays with Morrie* (Albom, 1997). There was no known cure for or even alleviation of the loss of muscular ability associated with the disease.

one that was charted by the life lessons I had learned while caring for my mother during this time. Although my primary interests had seemed to lie in the arts, after my mother's death I felt the need to answer a lingering call to service by becoming a nurse. Within 2 weeks of her death, I was enrolled in the nursing program at The University of Tennessee, Memphis, with no idea how it would turn out. The admissions interviewer asked me why I wanted to enter nursing. I told her I was interested in learning more about illness and disease, but that I wasn't sure I wanted to **do** anything about it. She suggested that maybe I should go into medicine.

I now find her response ironic, because the gist of medicine, the dominant emphasis on cure of disease, is the direction that I have found troublesome in the health-care system. This is not meant to be critical of medical science, just cognizant that its knowledge and focus are limited. What is needed is an understanding of health that encompasses the whole person, including disease. Medical practitioners are doing their share of the task of alleviating the burdens of disease, but there is a need for a shift from the narrow focus of eliminating the problem to the more inclusive perspective of helping people recognize the meaning of their lives when disease occurs.

Nursing is in a good position to facilitate this shift in the concept of health. But by having aligned ourselves with medicine, we have incorporated the value of curing and are reluctant to shift our focus to a more holistic perspective, even when it is clear that the cure objective cannot be met. From our very origin, nurses have been committed to a spiritual embrace of the one who is wounded or ill. *Caring* for the patient has been uppermost in nursing's mission. But caring alone has not been enough. We have to embrace a new vision of health. Our caring must be linked with a concept of health *that encompasses and goes beyond disease*. The *theory of health as expanding consciousness* provides that perspective.

The foundation of the theory was my lived experience as family caregiver. The relevancy of movement, space, and time as encountered in my prenursing experience, found new meaning as I studied rehabilitation nursing in graduate work at New York University and Rusk Institute in New York City. Restriction of movement was a factor in the quality of interpersonal relationships and the boundaries of patients' lives. My dissertation was an attempt to understand how variations in movement were related to one's experience of time (Newman, 1972).[2] The demands of the scientific method, however, were such that I tried to impose control on the natural human abilities to adjust to changing circumstances, and the results contributed very little to the understanding I was seeking for nursing practice situations. As I realized how participants in the study had compensated for the imposed alteration of their movement, I turned to the concept of consciousness as the important dimension to explore.

Itzhak Bentov's (1977, 1978) concept of expanding consciousness provided a breakthrough in my understanding of this phenomenon. Bentov's overarching thesis was that *life is the process of expanding consciousness.* He defined consciousness as the informational capacity of the system, as seen in the quality and quantity of interaction with the environment. He asserted that time is an index of consciousness.[3] When applied to the data of my early studies, this index revealed evidence of the expansion of consciousness across the life span (Newman, 1982). Evolving consciousness, a unitary concept, became the focus of the theory.

When asked to present my theory of nursing to a large conference of nursing educators, I relied on what I knew about movement, time, space, and consciousness (Newman, 1978). I had already incorporated Rogers' basic assumptions of wholeness, pattern, and unidirectionality in my thinking. My experience with my mother during her illness convinced me that the human being is unitary and that health encompasses and transcends disease. The basic assumptions of the theory, as articulated at that time (Newman, 1979), were:

1. *Health encompasses conditions heretofore described as illness, or in medical terms, pathology.*
   A person who has a pathological condition is not necessarily "ill." Experience with persons incapacitated in various ways by

---

[2]Participants in this experimental study were asked to estimate a short interval of time while walking at three speeds: personal tempo (PT), 30% faster than PT, and 30% slower than PT. Differences in time estimate were not significant, purportedly related to the participants' ability to compensate for the variation in movement.

[3]Bentov's index of consciousness consists of the ratio of subjective time (the participant's estimate) to objective time (as measured by the clock). For example, if one thinks 4 seconds have elapsed, but according to the clock, only 1 second has elapsed, the ratio would be 4:1 with a resulting index of consciousness of 4. When this index was calculated for data on persons of different age groups, the index ranged from .93 (mean age of 23) to 1.29 (mean age of 28) to 2.35 (mean age of 71).

chronic disease reveals that, for the most part, these people do not consider themselves sick. They may be unable to walk or to care for themselves, but from their point of view, they are not sick, unless perhaps they are inconvenienced by the common cold. As a matter of fact, nearly everyone of adult age has some condition that could be specified as pathological, with varying degrees of incapacitation, but each person is still very much a whole person.

2. *These "pathological" conditions can be considered a manifestation of the total pattern of the individual.*

   This statement is based on Rogers' (1970) earlier assumption that "Pattern and organization identify man [sic] and reflect his innovative wholeness" (p. 65). The story of my friend's experience with hyperthyroidism (see Introduction) illustrates this assumption. The pattern that is manifested in disease may be regarded as a clue to what is going on in the person's life, the dynamics of which the person may be unaware and cannot communicate in any other way.

3. *The pattern of the individual that eventually manifests itself as pathology is primary and exists prior to structural or functional changes.*

   An illustration of this point was suggested by Bahnson and Bahnson's (1966) theory of the rhythms of cancer. They maintained that the person who develops cancer manifests a pattern of very controlled interaction with the environment and uncontrolled internal processes. If this theory holds, the pattern exists before evidence of the cancer; the cancer is simply a manifestation of the pattern.[4]

4. *Removal of the pathology in itself will not change the pattern of the individual.*

   The underlying pattern will not be changed by simply eliminating the disease (the outward manifestation). Disease is something to be understood and experienced as a message. It can be an integrating factor, and as such, is important in the evolutionary process of the person.

---

[4]Later, Bohm's (1980) theory of implicate order lent support to this assumption. Bohm posited an underlying, unseen pattern, the implicate order, which exists before its explication in perceptible form.

5. *If becoming "ill" is the only way an individual's pattern can manifest itself, then that is health for that person.*

Illness, as an integrating factor, may accomplish for the person what she or he was unable to do otherwise. Stone (1978), a Jungian psychologist, pointed out that in his practice he doesn't keep track of people getting well anymore. Not that he is not pleased when someone does "get well," and not that feeling well is an unimportant consideration, but it is not of such importance that it is sought to the exclusion of the higher purpose of expanding consciousness.

The following statement was offered as the thesis of this approach:

Health is the expansion of consciousness.

Health is viewed as the totality of the life process, which is evolving toward expanded consciousness (Bentov, 1977).[5] The direction of evolution within the individual person, as well as within the species of mankind, is toward a realm of greater diversity and inclusiveness. This framework provides a view of health as the totality of the life process; therefore, one that encompasses disease as a meaningful aspect.

At the end of my presentation in 1978, I was asked to share my perspective on the goal of nursing. Based on these assumptions, I offered the conclusion that the goal of nursing is not to make people well, or to prevent their getting sick, but to assist them in using the power within as they evolve toward higher levels of consciousness. The audience response affirmed this direction for nursing.

AN OVERVIEW OF THE THEORY OF HEALTH AS EXPANDING CONSCIOUSNESS

The theory of health as expanding consciousness (HEC) was stimulated by my concern for those for whom health as the absence of disease or

---

[5]Bentov's (1977) definition of consciousness, the informational capacity of the system, includes all systems, from inanimate objects such as rocks, through all levels of plants and animals, to humans and beyond. Plants, for instance, have a consciousness (informational capacity) that interacts with the sun and seeks nourishment from the environment. Animals, with the added informational capacity of movement, have a greater ability to interact with the environment. The informational capacity of the human level goes beyond previous levels and includes all the physiological subsystems as well as the cognitive and affective abilities we normally associate with consciousness. According to Bentov, the consciousness of all systems interpenetrate; so we are always connected to and communicating with the whole of the universe.

disability is not possible. It has been extended to include persons in all health situations. Nurses often relate to people facing the uncertainty and loss associated with chronic illness and other disruptive forces in their lives. This theory asserts that every person in every situation, no matter how disordered and hopeless it may seem, is part of a process of expanding consciousness—a process of becoming more of oneself, of finding greater meaning in life, and of reaching new heights of connectedness with other people and the world.

Rogers' insistence that health and illness are simply manifestations of the rhythmic fluctuations of the life process led me to view health and illness as a unitary process. A familiar phenomenon that illustrates the unitary nature of life is body temperature. Body temperature fluctuates over a 24-hour period above and below what is labeled "normal" without being labeled pathological. The pattern of life also moves through peaks and troughs, variations in order-disorder that are meaningful for the person. From this standpoint, one can no longer think of health as dichotomous with disease, or even as a continuum from wellness to illness.[6] Health and the evolving pattern of consciousness are the same. This perspective recognizes consciousness as a creative process and focuses on health as a dialectical process between person and environment, as revealed in the dialogue between the health practitioner and the client (Litchfield, 1999).

The basic assumptions of the theory have been synthesized as follows:

- ■ Health is an evolving *unitary pattern* of the whole, including patterns of disease.
- ■ Consciousness is the *informational capacity* of the whole and is revealed in the evolving pattern.
- ■ Pattern identifies the human-environmental process and is characterized by *meaning*.

SUPPORTING THEORY

The theory of HEC is supported by the thinking of others, including prominently David Bohm's theory of implicate order, Ilya Prigogine's

---

[6]A continuum still polarizes the concept. If one moves toward one end, it is away from the other, meaning movement toward wellness diminishes illness, and vice versa.

theory of dissipative structures, and Arthur Young's theory of the evolution of consciousness.

Bohm's theory of implicate order (Bohm, 1980) supports the position of disease as a manifestation of the pattern of the whole. Bohm posited an unseen, underlying pattern as the primary order of reality; he called this the implicate order. All the tangible things of the world are explications of the implicate order. Thus, the explicate order is secondary to the implicate order. Information of the implicate order is present everywhere; it is not bound by space and time. It is available to us through our feelings via a resonant field (See Chapter 4). Disease, and all other observable manifestations of human functioning, can be seen as the explication of an underlying pattern. From this perspective, disease is considered a manifestation of the wholeness of the underlying pattern, not a separate entity.

The implicate order is fundamentally about processes in the non-energetic sense (Hiley, 2002). If we start with the implicate process, space-time will emerge from it as a kind of explicate order. The energy or activity that is there in the process is formless until a "thing" is formed. The subtle and the manifest form a unity, which constitutes consciousness. The highest level of consciousness is timeless and space-less: all time is at the present moment and all space is at each point in space.

Ilya Prigogine's theory of dissipative structures (Prigogine, 1976; Prigogine & Stengers, 1984) supports the assertion that even seemingly negative events, such as disease, are part of the process of expanding consciousness. According to Prigogine, a system fluctuates in an orderly manner until the occurrence of a disruptive event (internal and/or external), at which time the system moves in self-organizing but seemingly random, disorderly ways until it chooses a new direction at a higher level of organization. The disorder, if seen within the total context, is a pathway to higher consciousness.

Arthur Young (1976) offered a theory of the evolution of consciousness elaborating stages of the process of expanding consciousness, especially evident at the nadir choice point at which the old ways are not working, and a shift in perspective must occur. A person moves through stages of consciousness involving the loss of freedom in the development of self-identity until a turning point is reached when the "old rules" don't work anymore. The life task is to discover the "new rules" and make a choice that allows greater freedom and sensitivity and goes beyond the limitations of an objective space-time world, moving toward increasing freedom and higher consciousness. Characteristic of this latter trajectory is an involvement in matters greater than the individual self (Newman, 1994).

The information of the human system (consciousness) is in the form of a dynamic pattern. Consistent with Bohm's theory of implicate order, Whitmont (1994), a Jungian physician, has taken the position that each person has an innate and intrinsic force, like having an essential dynamic purpose, underlying the unfolding of an individual's pattern. It may be expected to guide transformation, because it is inherent in human nature to grow and change: *"It may . . . even be bent upon imbalancing and upsetting an existing state of health if and when this state no longer accords with the growth needs of the total personality.* This 'wounding or partial destruction' corresponds to the paradox expressed by Apollo that 'that which wounds shall also heal'"* (p. 13, emphasis added). Whitmont related this correspondence to Jung's assertion of the drive to fulfill one's wholeness of life pattern, to become what one is, to explicate the guidance of the implicate order. These assertions support the position that disease be looked upon as a manifestation of expanding consciousness. The information of the implicate order is not material but may utilize materiality and have material effects.

How does the unitary, transformative paradigm influence practice? Disease is no longer the primary focus. The focus is on the person, the pattern of the evolving whole, of transformations within transformations, including the unpredictability of chaotic systems. This new order has new rules. One of them, perhaps the foremost, is the necessity of unconditional love, which manifests itself in sensitivity to self, attention to others, and creativity. This is what we seek for our clients and for ourselves.

DEVELOPMENT OF THE THEORY THROUGH RESEARCH

Based on the assumption that disease is a manifestation of the pattern of the whole, I initiated a program of research to examine the major thesis of health as expanding consciousness with participants who had been diagnosed with various chronic diseases. The objective was to understand the underlying, unfolding pattern of their lives by asking them to tell about the most meaningful relationships and events in their lives.[7] Their stories revealed the important relationships in their unfolding patterns, and began to point the way toward understanding the evolving process.

In developing a method of research that was consistent with the theory of HEC, I settled on the descriptors hermeneutic and dialectic: hermeneutic to denote the search for meaning and understanding through interpretation, and dialectic because both the process of the method (between researcher and participant) and the content of the search (the participant's interaction with others) were dialectic (Newman, 1994). The method allows the pattern of person-environment to reveal itself without disturbing the unity of the pattern. The process culminates in intuitive apprehension and expression. The practitioner-researcher (PR) enters into a dialectic relationship with the client-participant (CP), especially when the CP is experiencing disruption and uncertainty. A reflective dialogue centering on the meaningfulness of the CP's pattern of relationships is maintained during the period of uncertainty until insight occurs and the CP's pattern shifts to a higher order. (See Appendix A)

Elements of the practice/research process are: establishing the mutuality of the process, focusing on the most meaningful events and relationships in the CP's life, viewing the CP's story as an unfolding pattern, and sharing the PR's perception of the pattern with the CP. The relationship is characterized by receptivity, reciprocity, and a feeling of oneness. Inherent in the process is the insight CPs gain as the pattern is discerned, and with it, the illumination and activation of action possibilities. Timing of the PR-CP encounter in the overall scheme of things may be important. The process appears to progress more rapidly when the CP is in a particularly disruptive situation.

A shift in the nature of the research and a clearer understanding of the nurse-client relationship occurred upon Litchfield's (1999) insistence that the focus of pattern recognition should be the *process* of the evolving pattern, rather than the pattern itself. The process **is** the content. Along with other parameters of the scientific method, the PR had to let go of prediction and control as necessary elements. The PR was integral to the process, as was the embodied theory. The evolving relationship of PR and CP was making a difference in both their lives. The PR

---

[7]After several attempts to identify pattern by asking specific questions regarding movement, space, and time, Susan Moch, my research assistant at the time, said "I'd just like to ask them to tell me about the most meaningful experience in their life. That made sense to me, and it has proved to be a fruitful way to stimulate the storytelling that reveals life pattern.

could not stand apart as an objective observer. The PR had to become comfortable with letting go of control and living with the uncertainty of unpredictability in the process. At the same time, the PR was not an "empty" bystander, but responded in a knowledgeable manner. The focus on the evolving pattern of the client emphasized what is meaningful to the client and enhanced an understanding of nursing practice. The dynamic nature of the process, and the instantaneous difference that arose in the lives of both the clients and the nurses, revealed the nature of the research itself as transformative practice. In practice, the thrust of the pattern may become apparent quickly as an observation, an intuitive metaphor, or repeated complaint. For example, Margaret Pharris (personal communication) was referred to a man who had sought medical help repeatedly for chest pain to no avail. Her response to his complaint was, "Your heart must be hurting (aching)," to which he shared the heartbreak of his wife's having left him and what that meant to him. Acknowledgment by the practitioner to the client opens the way for further elaboration, insight, and action.

The emphasis of this process is on knowing/caring through pattern recognition. This type of relationship has no specific prescriptive component. As the interpenetration of the fields of two or more persons occurs, the participants resonate with the information of the field, the pattern is clarified, and the CPs experience insight regarding actions they may take. This experience is a dynamic interface of theory, research, and practice, that is, praxis. The theory guides the inquiry and makes a difference in the lives of the participants; in turn, the data of the process elaborates the theory. That kind of knowledge is needed in nursing.

The shift from a problem orientation to *pattern* recognition is a shift to a higher dimension of knowledge, one that includes and transcends all that has gone before. Pattern depicts relationships and pulls it all together. Opposites fade away in the overall scheme of things. Dichotomies no longer exist. Parts are permeated by the pattern of the whole and become a way of seeing the whole. Dorothy Jones (personal communication) pointed out that, "The integration of a method that calls forth the story, the process which guides the emergence of the story, and the theory which frames the nursepatient[8] relationship offer new vision—a new way to approach nursing."

---

[8]From time to time, the terms "patient" and "client" are used interchangeably as a matter of the author's preference. I trust the reader will understand the ambiguity of the way we in nursing regard the focus of our practice.

Chapter 2

Shifting to a
New Paradigm

*Do you know where you were when the
paradigm shifted?*

Marilyn Ferguson, Circa 1983

erhaps the most dramatic paradigm shift in modern history is attributed to Copernicus. Through years of study he was able to
point out that the earth and other planets revolved around the
sun, rather than the other way around. This new knowledge was revolutionary and changed the world's thinking about the universe. It's important to recognize that he was looking at the same elements but *seeing
them differently*. Once that view was validated, there was no going back.

THE SHIFT IN THE PERSPECTIVE OF HEALTH

A major shift has been occurring in the health field: from a focus on disease to a focus on *pattern* and *health* (Ferguson, 1980). This perspective
has been evident in nursing since the days of Nightingale (1859), who
saw disease as a reparative process and pointed out that the laws of
health were the same for the "well as among the sick" (p. 6). Rogers
(1970) confirmed this view as the foundation of nursing with her emphasis on wholeness and pattern. The shift is from treatment of symptoms of disease to a search for patterns; from viewing pain and disease as
wholly negative to viewing them as information about the pattern of
the whole; from seeing the body as a machine in good or bad repair to

11

seeing the person as a dynamic field continuous with the larger environmental field; from seeing disease as an separate entity to seeing it as a unitary process.

The theory of health as expanding consciousness (Newman, 1978; 1979; 1986; 1994) reflects this shift within nursing with an emphasis on the meaningfulness of the pattern as a whole. When Flanagan (2005) introduced this shift to the nursing staff in a preadmission surgical clinic, they were able to see the surgical experience in the center of the whole of the patient's experience. For example, one nurse was able to help a patient see her illness-experience as a symbol of the blocking of her own passion and creativity, and the removal of the offending organ as an opportunity to bring creativity back into her life.

This paradigm of health assumes an underlying connecting pattern, such as Bohm's theory of implicate order (Bohm, 1980) and Bateson's metapattern, the pattern that connects (Bateson, 1979). The nature of the identifying pattern is consciousness: the total informational capacity of the system, the ability of the system to interact with the larger system. Consciousness and matter are manifestations of the same underlying pattern. One does not precede the other. Just as matter and energy are different manifestations of the same underlying phenomenon, so our physical being and the aspects of ourselves we associate with mind are different manifestations of the same underlying pattern. The process of life, that is, health, is a process of expanding consciousness. This unitary process moves through periods of order and disorder, harmony and disharmony, calm and crisis, wellness and illness.

The shift is occurring in medicine as well:

> "Health is seen not as the absence of disease, but as a process by which individuals maintain their ability to develop a meaning system that will allow them to function in the face of changes in themselves and their relationships with their environment" (Schlitz, Taylor, and Lewis, 1998, p. 48).
>
> "While science has contributed to our understanding and treatment of disease, it has also served to limit the development of a model in which personal relationships, emotions, meaning, and belief systems are viewed as fundamental points of connection between body, mind, spirit, society, and the environment. For increasing numbers of healthcare consumers and professionals alike, the biomedical model fails to offer a system for understanding the fullness of lived experience—minimizing or negating completely the possibility for human transcendence in the face of illness and disease" (Schlitz, 2004, p. 8).

Shostak and Whitehouse (1999), who referred to the diseases of today as diseases of meaning, suggested that awareness of the process could shift a person's perspective to enable him or her to see disease as a manifestation of health. Miles (1998), a spokesman for the holistic health movement at the Institute of Noetic Sciences, referred to healing as a shift in personal perspective rather than a rescue. Grossinger (2004) viewed illness as an integral part of who we are and healing as a reconciliation with the superordinate pattern of the world.

What are the essential characteristics of this paradigm? One is that there is increasing *uncertainty* (Paul, Akers, Dunn, and Brodsky, 1986). Nursing researcher Mishel's (1990) conceptualization of uncertainty corresponds to Prigogine's (1976) period of disorganization as the sequel to coping with uncertainty, which is viewed as an opportunity to make a transition from one perspective of life to another at a higher order. In contrast, when we are convinced we know what will happen next, based on past experience or empirical evidence, we may be closed to alternative possibilities. There is no way to predict the evolutionary unfolding before all of the factors come into play. For example, uncertainty can be experienced in atonal music with its clusters of arrhythmic bursts. One cannot anticipate the next tone or rhythm. One must be fully present in the moment. The intensity of uncertainty pierces straight through to one's feelings; it is not an intellectual activity. People usually foreclose on uncertainty to avoid the experience of disequilibrium, which is an aspect of growth. Learning is often painful; the input to the system is greater than one's processing ability. The creative act occurs at extreme disequilibrium when one is moving on to something unknown (Thompson, 1991). Transition to the unknown is difficult.

The order of the new paradigm is a *dynamic order:* a process (Goodwin, 1991) and an ordering principle (Goethe, in Bortoft, 1996). The whole organism as the fundamental entity in biology generates parts that conform to an intrinsic order, a unity. The order is revealed in the relationships that emerge. This paradigm requires that we study the organism in a way that does not fragment its unity, a way that allows the organism to speak to us without disturbing its state. The system is always in process. In nursing, the focus of our study is the nursing relationship with person/family/community that must be allowed to reveal itself without interruption.

The paradigm shift is apparent in nursing research. Recognizing the ongoing conflict among nursing scientists regarding the value of different forms of research, my colleagues and I sought to explain the conflict from the standpoint of philosophy of science by identifying the different rules guiding the prevailing paradigms of nursing research (Newman,

Sime, and Corcoran-Perry, 1991). As we saw it, nursing research could be identified as emanating from the standpoint of three perspectives:[1]

1. Particulate-deterministic: From this perspective, variables can be isolated, controlled, manipulated, and predicted. Causal inference can be made. Experimental conditions simulate a treatment mode; that is, something can be employed to hypothesize a specific effect.
2. Interactive-integrative: In this mode, the researcher is still an outside observer with the intent but not the ability to control the variables. It stems from a social interactive perspective and takes into account multiple variables with some predictability.
3. Unitary-transformative: Here a major shift has occurred. The researcher is a participant in the evolving pattern of the whole. There is an inability to separate parts (variables); therefore, an inability to control and predict. Change comes about as transformation of the total pattern.

It was our intent to give equal emphasis to each of the paradigms, but by the time we had finished our analysis and explication, we were aware that the unitary-transformative (UT) perspective represented a dramatic shift in paradigm that was crucial in the development of nursing knowledge. Similarly, Parse's (1987) explication of the simultaneity paradigm represents an irreversible shift to a unitary view. The emphasis on a unitary view, introduced by Rogers (1970), was a major turning point in the development of nursing knowledge. It does not preclude recognition of knowledge emanating from the other paradigms but presents, as in the Copernican shift, a totally new view, one that is seen as essential to knowledge development in nursing (Newman, 1997). Phillips (1990, p. 103) described the change:

> Research should focus on elucidating how changes in health situations emerge from this mutual process. This requires nurse researchers to move their focus of study from illness and disease to health, their sense of interconnectedness with others, and specifically how health[2] emerges from a mutual process.

Explication of the differences in nursing paradigms has created the misconception of competing realms of knowledge. The paradigms were

---

[1]The first word in each pairing represents the nature of the phenomenon. The second word denotes the nature of the change that occurs.
[2]One's concept of health is important here.

described individually but were not intended to represent separate knowledge; the delineation was simply an attempt to explain differing views of nursing and the human experience. There was an intuitive recognition of the evolution of theory related to nursing from particulate to reciprocal to unitary ways of knowing. This recognition was clouded by our need to respect each type of theory and to give equal time and credence to each body of work. In actuality, we were seeing the UT view emerging as inclusive of the previous foci: including and transcending that which has gone before.

How can we deal with contradictory points of view? Just as relativity theory can include mechanistic theory as special cases, the unitary perspective can include the more particulate view. A three-dimensional perspective (length, width, and height) includes a two-dimensional perspective (length and width), but the Flatlander, an inhabitant of a flat two-dimensional world (Abbott, 1952), cannot imagine the world of three dimensions. If a balloon invades his territory, it comes across as merely a circle of varying sizes as it passes through. In the same way, the practitioner limited to a particulate view of phenomena will be unable to grasp the more complex unitary view.

The growth in understanding has been evolutionary. We first thought of the different paradigms as standing alone, but now recognize the common ground of the more inclusive UT world view. Nursing knowledge is a process of the patterning of the whole. It is important that the practitioner of nursing incorporate the knowledge of earlier realms as special cases of the pattern of the whole. For example, a nurse, while attending to the meaning a patient ascribes to falling at a particularly critical time in her or his life, will at the same time apply ice packs to prevent swelling in the injured parts. Knowledge of traumatic injury is relevant in this situation, as well as knowledge of the whole.

The paradox is that there are no boundaries between paradigms. Delineating the paradigms was done to facilitate understanding of the rules of the game. Unitary-transformative approaches cannot be held to the criteria of control and prediction; and research conducted in the particulate-deterministic perspective is not adequate to the task of illuminating the meaning of the emerging pattern of a nurse-client relationship. But knowledge from both approaches can be incorporated in practice, which includes and transcends all knowledge.

The participatory nature of the UT paradigm is crucial. Skolimowski (1994) pointed out that in the dynamic reality of increasing complexity and expanding consciousness, there must be an accompanying thread of simplicity and comprehension. This is how the participatory nature of the nurse in pattern recognition makes the difference in the client's experience of *insight,* which is moving and relational and involves recognition of things going on (Briggs & Peat, 1990). The skill of the nurse in facilitating this understanding is related to the level of consciousness of the nurse. The seemingly simple question, "Tell me about the most meaningful experiences in your life" (See Appendix A), opens a world of complexity that reveals the pattern of a person's life and with it the transformative insight that shifts her or his worldview. The nurse must be fully present in this process. From Skolimowski (1994, p. 151): "The degree, depth and richness of our participation determines the richness and meaningfulness of our life. Those who for one reason or another refuse to participate impoverish their lives," and, I would add, the lives of those whom they serve.

This new kind of knowledge requires a transition from objective consciousness to compassionate consciousness (similar to Watson's [1999] caring consciousness), a kind of participation "that compassionately embraces the other, that dwells in the other, that tries to understand the other from within" (Skolimowski, 1994, p. 174). It does not deny objective thinking; it transcends it. The more meaningful the participation, the more truth it reveals. The path of participatory knowledge is sometimes messy; those who follow the path of absolute knowledge appear to be more secure, but the latter is static and without novelty.

Acceptance of the essential nature of the UT paradigm would be a giant step in unifying the nursing profession. We could then be more specific about the nature of theory-guided[3] practice. Nursing theory is a point of view (Donaldson & Crowley, 1978). It determines how one views the client and environment, how one views the role of a nurse, and how one views health. These views constitute a paradigm of nursing knowledge, and nursing knowledge focuses on relating to people in their health experience. The literature supports the focus of nursing as *caring in the human health experience* (Newman, Sime, and Corcoran-Perry, 1991). From the standpoint of the theory of HEC, one views the client and environment as unitary, evolving patterns; the role of the nurse as a caring, pattern-recognizing presence; and health as a transformative process to more inclusive consciousness.

---

[3] Not to be confused with evidence-based practice.

THE SHIFT IN THE STUDY OF CONSCIOUSNESS

Parallel to shifts in the health field was Willis Harman's challenge to the scientific paradigm in the study of consciousness (Harman, 1988). When Harman was president of the Institute of Noetic Sciences, an organization devoted to the study of consciousness, he initiated a dialogue with leading scientists in the field of consciousness about the inadequacy of the traditional scientific paradigm for the study of consciousness. As background, he stated his beliefs that every person has a deep sense of purpose, that we need to learn to create a vision, and that we need to cultivate a particular attitude regarding our actions; that is, to welcome feedback even if it is in the form of failure, opposition, and so on, and learn from it because it is all part of the deep intuitive purpose of the universe. He reiterated points from perennial wisdom that the universe can be trusted and that the deep intuition of the universe has a role for the individual in its evolutionary drama. In his view, the universe is saturated with purpose. These views are consistent with Tarnas' (1998) understanding of the history of knowledge development and are relevant to nursing science.

Harman began his explication of a new paradigm in which consciousness, rather than the matter-energy of the positivist-reductionist approach, is the basic stuff of the universe and is primary: "Ultimately reality is contacted not through the senses but through deep intuition" (Harman, 1988). Intuition is an important dimension of knowing and reveals the unity of the pattern that is missed by the intellectual mind.

By 1993, Harman had developed an epistemology of consciousness, endorsed by 19 other leading scholars in the field, which was a sharp contrast to the positivist-reductionist approach. In contrast to modern science's attempt to control bias by excluding the observer, Harman pointed out that in consciousness research, neither the researcher nor the researched is more objective than the other, that they are collaborators at the same level. Selected points of the new epistemology were (Harman, 1993, pp. 75–76):

■ It is experiential in nature and includes subjective experience as primary data. It addresses the totality of human experience. "Thus, consciousness is not a 'thing' to be studied by an observer who is somehow apart from it; consciousness involves the *interaction* of the observer and the observed, or, if you like, the *experience* of observing" (p. 75).

- ▪ It will aim at being objective in the sense of being open and free from hidden bias while dealing with both external and internal experience as origins of data.
- ▪ It will insist on open inquiry and public validation of knowledge, but may not be able to meet this goal completely.
- ▪ It will place emphasis upon the *unity* of experience. ". . . the meanings of experiences may be understood by discovering their interconnections with other meaningful experiences" (p. 76).
- ▪ It will be *participatory*. This implies partnership between the researcher and the individual or culture being researched—an attitude of exploring together and sharing understandings.
- ▪ It will recognize the inescapable role of the personal characteristics of the observer; therefore, the researcher "must **be willing to risk being profoundly changed** through the process . . ." (emphasis in original, p. 76).
- ▪ Because of the potential transformation of the observers, the epistemology may be replaced by more enlightened practices.

THE STUDY OF HEALTH AS EXPANDING CONSCIOUSNESS (HEC)

Harman's assertions regarding the study of consciousness lent support to an experiential, participatory approach to the study of HEC. As I searched for an appropriate methodology for studying the theory of health as expanding consciousness, I went from experimental (Newman, 1972) to quasiexperimental (Newman & Gaudiano, 1984) to finally letting go of the old rules and establishing a process of mutuality in looking at the evolving pattern of persons facing major health problems (Newman, 1987). Based on an appreciation for the unitary nature of the nurse-client encounter, the process began with attention to meaning in the client/participant's life. Pattern recognition occurred in the process as clients began to sense intuitively the pattern of their lives, and with it an emerging insight regarding action to be taken and an openness to more caring relationships in their lives.

I now realize that the development of nursing knowledge is not scientific in the traditional sense. Goodwin (1991) suggested that eventually we can drop the term science altogether and just talk of knowledge, with no need to separate art and science. The development of nursing knowledge occurs as the process of nursing praxis. The focus of the discipline of nursing is a relational activity in regard to the client's health. In this process, one cannot separate the observer from the observed and cannot control the multiple factors involved in the situation. It is necessary to embrace the unitary nature of the process in its totality and allow the pattern to unfold. The emphasis has moved from observation of the pattern of the other to the relational process of the nurse and client. If one is looking for outcomes based on the theory, they will be found in the clients' understanding of their life patterns and actions that reveal transformation to more meaningful relationships. Research that only names, that is describes, a phenomenon in an observer-observed mode does not reflect the dialectic process of the knowledge that is nursing. Research that controls and predicts relates to another paradigm.

Goodwin (1991, p. 15), speaking from the standpoint of a biologist, suggested a replacement of a historical, reductionistic paradigm of events by a generative paradigm of process: ". . . the whole problem . . . is to learn how to hold this totality in mind . . . to reveal the type of dynamic order there is in organisms—the real generative order." The pattern of the whole is the order that directs the development of the parts. Goodwin called for a way to study organisms without fragmenting their unity, to allow the organism to speak without disrupting its states. One of his observations that is particularly relevant to the human situation is that ". . . organisms . . . *must change in order to be themselves*, have to constantly move and transform"(p. 18, emphasis added). He, too, with Harman, pointed out that as we incorporate new knowledge, we ourselves are transformed.

With the paradigm shift in nursing, new vision regarding knowledge development is required. The concept of praxis, having been framed by the ideological movements related to class, race, and gender, is nevertheless fitting for nursing. The knowledge of our discipline must be theory-based, subjected to a form of inquiry, and practice-relevant. The predominant theories in nursing embrace values inherent in the profession: wholeness (health), caring, evolving pattern, mutual process, and transformation. The phenomenon of nursing is a dynamic nurse-client relationship viewed within a unitary perspective of health. The merging of theory, research, and practice, as in praxis, is appropriate for knowledge and practice development in the discipline.

Chapter 3

Nursing Praxis

The theory is the practice.

—Virginia A. Capasso, 2005

In nursing praxis, research takes the form of practice. It involves specific nurse-client relationships in situations of concern to nursing. Nursing praxis includes and transcends the nursing knowledge of our past. The focus of nursing praxis includes both personal and environmental systems; it integrates knowledge from other disciplines. From the standpoint of health as expanding consciousness (HEC), nursing praxis is:

- Grounded in a unitary, transformative paradigm.
- A dynamic partnership between nurse and client.
- A dialogue of an evolving pattern of meaning, insight, and action.
- Transforming for both nurse and client.

HEC praxis represents a shift in knowledge development from a rational, logical, objective approach to an intuitive, resonant, unitary approach. It makes a difference in people's lives. Nursing praxis is a mutual process between nurse and client with the intent to help. It focuses on transformation from one point to another and incorporates the guidance of a priori theory. It involves the intersection between the client's self-understanding and the researcher's embodied theoretical perspective. The theory illuminates the experience, which in turn illuminates the theory.

One definition of praxis is that it "enables people to change by encouraging self-reflection and a deeper understanding of their particular situations" (Lather, 1986, p. 263). One of the premises of HEC is that insight into pattern illuminates the potential for action for both the client and the practitioner. Endo, Miyahara, Suzuki, and Ohmasa (2005) reported that practicing nurses who followed the praxis protocol for pattern recognition (Newman, 1994) found that "most patients changed quickly in the process of talking [about] themselves. Some patients made big transformations. The turning point for the nurses appeared after they had realized the patients' change."

The theory of health as expanding consciousness embodies the practice of nursing, and when combined with systematic inquiry, constitutes nursing praxis. The research component centers on pattern recognition, but must be characterized by the caring relatedness of the nurse-patient partnership. Some of the published studies emphasize the pattern identified for the clients, whereas others are more explicit about the process of the nurse-client relationship. The pattern becomes apparent as clients tell their stories of meaningful persons and events in their lives. Feedback to the client by diagram, narrative, and/or other portrayals facilitates revelation of the pattern and with it, the transformation apparent in intuitive bursts of insight and action. In addition to focusing on the client's most meaningful experiences, Pharris (2002) elaborated the nurse-client relationship that is key to the process:

> Nurses practicing from the HEC perspective attend to the physical manifestations and patterns of interaction of their patients to sense the implicate pattern. An HEC nurse develops multifaceted levels of awareness to be able to sense the underlying pattern in a person's physical appearance and symptoms, emotional conveyances, spiritual insights, mental ponderings, tone of voice, movements, etc. The reflective nature of the HEC nurse-client relationship facilitates pattern recognition. HEC nursing involves being fully present to the client without judgments, goals, or intervention strategies. It entails *being with* rather than *doing for*. It forms a partnership that involves caring in its deepest, most respectful sense. It is in the context of the nurse-client relationship that pattern can be recognized; as this happens, action potential arises and transformation becomes a possibility (p. 23).

How the nurse facilitates pattern recognition is more important than enumerating the patterns that evolve. Each nursing encounter will be different and what practicing nurses must learn is how to be fully present in the moment of encounter with the client. The phases of the process have been identified as moving through (1) establishing the mutuality of the initial encounter, (2) evolving dialogue and pattern recognition, and (3) experiencing insight, transformation, and action at a more inclusive, caring level of consciousness (Endo, 1998; Litchfield, 1999; Shields & Lindsey, 1998). Where community health is the focus, the reciprocal of individual and family patterns may be identified and shared with community participants by various forms of group presentation for feedback regarding its relevance to their community (Pharris, 2005). An overview of some of the praxis studies follows.

PATTERNS OF INDIVIDUALS

The first HEC study, designed to identify patterns of persons with coronary heart disease (CHD) (Newman & Moch, 1991), revealed unique patterns that could be categorized according to Young's (1976) spectrum of evolving consciousness. Some of the participants were caught up in answering to the needs of others (binding stage); most were striving to establish their own identities (centering stage); and some were at the choice point of seeking a better way to live their lives. The important revelation for nursing knowledge was that the emphasis was on the *meaning* that the disruption of CHD had for each person. The things that were most meaningful to the participants were a sense of who they were, a need to develop better relationships with members of their family, and a desire to discover a new way of life. A nurse's presence opened the way to movement along the evolutionary spectrum. A similar study with persons diagnosed with cancer revealed patterns of deprivation in childhood and lack of connectedness throughout their lives. With the presence of a caring nurse, one participant in particular found new meaning in her sense of being cared for and in feeling her own warmth toward others (Newman, 1995).

A study of persons with HIV/AIDS supported the view of disease as a manifestation of expanding consciousness: "The loss of membranal integrity associated with HIV/AIDS opens the person to suffering and physical deterioration and at the same time introduces greater sensitivity and openness to self and others. The men in this study moved from being separated, alienated individuals in search of their place and connection in life to more meaningful, authentic relationships with self and others" (Lamendola & Newman, 1994, p. 20). The interviewing nurse's understanding of HEC made it possible for him to receive the paradoxical nature of the client/participant's pain and joy in such a way that they could be open to the whole of their experience.

Several investigators have chosen to relate to cancer patients: Endo (1998) conducted a study of pattern recognition with Japanese women who had ovarian cancer. As the women got in touch with their own patterns, the transformation that was occurring was observable as a "brightness" of their demeanor. Endo found that the women who were in situations of extreme disturbance moved along quickly to a point of insight and transformation. This factor was supported in subsequent studies; Kiser-Larson (2002), in her study of Native American women experiencing breast cancer, also found that the most opportune time for pattern recognition to occur was when the women were in a situation of turmoil.

Barron (2005) added to the support for growth and transformation in the midst of suffering. Participants in her study had cancer, and many were in near-death situations; yet they continued to flourish. She came to see end of life as a time of growth and possibility. Barron saw the process of identifying pattern as the essence of nursing practice: ". . . the nurse is fully present and participates in a transformational process as meaning unfolds" (p. 45). She reinforced the position that even though the patterns per se are meaningful, the more meaningful aspect of this HEC practice is the process of relationship with the participants and staff. She concluded, "I am changed by the wisdom and love they shared."

Studies of persons with chronic obstructive pulmonary disease in Iceland and in the United States yielded mixed results (Jonsdottir, 1998; Noveletsky-Rosenthal, 1996). The predominant pattern was one of isolation and lack of connectedness with other people, a pattern that mirrors the dynamics of their lung capacity. At the same time, some of the participants were able to sense into their pattern, make choices, and transcend the illness situation. As found in previous studies, the differentiating factor may have been the timing of the nursing encounter. If it occurred early in the diagnostic period (a time of high turbulence), the participants were more likely to respond to the pattern recognition process.

Neill's (2002a; 2002b) report of her partnership with Australian women who were living with multiple sclerosis and rheumatoid arthritis yielded stories of transcendence and transformation. She saw a clear role for nursing as making a difference in people's lives: "My work did not alter their [disease], for that is not the intention of unitary-transformative nursing, but it did make a difference in their lives. . . . my understanding of life patterns and underlying patterns indicated the potential for nursing in harmony with the individual rhythms and patterns; for the first time it allowed me to perceive the wholeness of the individuals" (2002a, p. 46). Neill asserted that one of the most important aspects of HEC is the mutual, caring relationship and dialogue that evolves within a nursing partnership. She acknowledged the difficulty (and importance) of tolerating uncertainty in the process but after a while found it liberating.

Rosa (2006) chose to work with persons living with chronic skin wounds (CSW). Insight into each participant's unique pattern as it relates to Young's stages of consciousness enhanced understanding that "human development of consciousness is an essential element in healing and recovery" (p. 352). The trajectory of participants' lives moved from deprivation during childhood through forging ahead in the face of pain and suffering to a significant loss, which preceded the manifestation of the CSW. With the help of a sensitive, caring nurse, participants began to recognize a new sense of self and personal awareness. "*Insight* occurred when a connection was made between a personal awareness around wound healing and a meaningful life" and "brought new energy and movement toward personal change" (p. 354). Rosa's model of healing focused on the whole person, not just the illness. Here is the way she described the process of healing:

> Participants integrated their problems, created deeper connections with others, and accelerated personal growth and healing. As one problem improved, awareness began to shift to other concerns needing attention, and the healing process repeated itself with another new awareness leading to greater transformation. . . . Guided by the nurse each participant identified unique and specific behaviors to enhance wound healing and enacted them (p. 357).

Several studies have focused on women's health. Picard (2000) led the way in relating to midlife women from nonclinical settings. She picked up on movement, one of the early parameters of wholeness in the theory of HEC, and incorporated creative movement as a way of expressing pattern. Berry (2004) followed with a study of women who were successful in maintaining weight loss. The parallels between the women's personal journeys and their progression on Young's spectrum of evolving consciousness were helpful in understanding the changes that took place. Musker (2005) chose women in transition through menopause as the focus of her HEC praxis. She identified the predominant level of consciousness for each participant and how their patterns were evolving to a higher stage. Most of the participants had reached the centering stage (Young, 1976). She pointed out the importance for the nurse to trust the process and wait in silence as the pattern surfaces.

FAMILY AND COMMUNITY

Continued research, relating not only to adults with medically diagnosed diseases, but also to other health-care crises in families and communities, highlighted the importance of the nursing relational process in reaching the insight that was a transforming factor. Litchfield's (1999) work in New Zealand illustrated the transforming difference the nurse's presence can make in families with children who had been repeatedly hospitalized. She coined the term "health dialectic" to describe the dialogic process of differing concepts of health within the practitioner-client partnership. She referred to her dialectical perspective on caring and health as practice wisdom. Tommet (2003), too, partnered with families of medically fragile children with the intent of examining their decision-making process related to choice of schooling. As the study unfolded, Tommet was able to assist the families in seeing the evolving trajectory of their lives in facing the uncertainty of their situation and learning to live and thrive in the present. Unfortunately the difficulties they struggled with were "made worse by conflicting confrontations with health, education and human service bureaucracies" (p. 246). Tommet's study called for a family-oriented approach, one that a knowledgeable, caring nurse could establish. Falkenstern's (2003) exploration of the nurse-client process in the emerging life patterns in families who have a child with special health-care needs emphasized the transformational experience of both the nurse and the clients as they struggled with the uncertainty and confusion of their situations.

Pharris (2002) chose to concentrate her focus on partnership with adolescents convicted of murder. Her study yielded three important findings: a description of the participants' pathway that preceded the murder and incarceration; an elaboration of the process of nurse-client pattern recognition and transformation as facilitated by the nurse; and the reciprocal community pattern with implications for action. Pharris' explication of the process of the nurse-client partnership revealed the isolation, abuse, and hurt of these adolescents and their disconnect from family, school, and legitimate community services. The alternative for their survival was alignment with gangs and drug dealers, which led to loss of a sense of self in the abuse of drugs and gun activity, which ultimately led to murder. Incarceration provided a respite, in a way, from the frantic street activity—an opportunity to slow down and begin to connect with self. Pharris' partnership with these adolescents was a transforming event in their lives.

Developing a trusting relationship was not easy for the young men in Pharris' study. It "was like being in a foreign land and not knowing the language or the culture" (p. 35). Some, who had suffered severe childhood abuse, had never known a relationship that was not filled with hate, drunkenness, and abuse. As participants were able to recognize and understand the pattern of their lives, there was "a deep level of connecting with their true selves" (p. 36). They began to feel their emotions, which had somehow been turned off for a long time. They began to relax and let go of the tough-guy demeanor. One participant referred to the revelation of finding himself as like finding buried treasure. The process of connecting to self became the potential for transforming action, such as engaging in further education. This study supports the transformative power of the nurse's partnership with these young men and reveals the lack of effective community support for the nurturance and guidance of young parents. The school, a potential crucial point of contact for both the parents and their children, somehow failed to maintain a connection with these lost adolescents. Pharris wrote: "Youth losing their connection to school is a health issue and nurses working within the school system can take leadership in assuring that the school system responds quickly and intensively to youth who do not show up for school. Truancy is a health issue in which nurses should be involved" (p. 40). Pharris concluded that HEC nursing "focuses more on a *way of being in relationship* than on measurement of effective actions for change" (p. 41). This is an important lesson to be learned in whatever practice setting nurses find themselves.

MODELS OF PRACTICE

The focus of HEC research was broadened to include models of practice. Eager to extend the transforming benefits of practice based on HEC, Endo and her colleagues conducted an action research project involving practicing nurses, revealing deepening meaning in the lives of the professional nurses as they experienced the transformative power of pattern recognition in their clients (Endo, Miyahara, et al., 2005). The nurses were hesitant at first to move beyond the established intent of "doing for" the clients to address problems of the disease, but found the clients eager to talk to them about what they found meaningful, and as the nurses witnessed the transformations taking place in the clients' lives, they too were transformed and released to engage more fully in the relationships with their clients: "Once the nurses captured the heart of the theory through experience, they could not forget what the clients' potential was like" (p. 144). They learned "that meaning in nursing situations was not *out there*, but was created in the client-nurse relationship as it was unfolding" (p. 144). This experience reinforced Endo's earlier assertion of this process as "a meaning-making-transformative process" (Endo, Nitta, et al., 2000, p. 609).

Flanagan (2005) recognized a need to distinguish the role of nurses from that of other health-care providers in a preadmission clinic. Her leadership with staff began with a shift in the philosophical and ontological beliefs about dimensions of person, health, nursing:

> Their prior views about person and disease had focused on illness as an obstacle to be overcome. As nurses began to shift from a disease model to a process model, . . . they became able to understand the patient experience from the stories told. What also became clear was that the individual's life was more than the surgical intervention. By restricting all conversation to the surgical event, nurses found they were not fully coming to know their patients or what the illness experience truly meant (p. 57).

As positive as these changes were for the patients, some of the nurses felt increasingly vulnerable in the open-ended, transformative nature of the process as compared with their previous circumscribed "expert" role as a technician. The authenticity of their own changes opened new uncertainties. As the nurses began to link to their new HEC perspective, they could see how their presence during the preop period helped to change the patient's experience; and patients expressed a desire for a continuing relationship with the nurse throughout their hospital stay.

Ruka (2005), in developing a new model of practice in a nursing home, took on the difficult task of pattern recognition with persons with dementia. These persons often have difficulty communicating verbally; therefore, pattern recognition was based primarily on observed behaviors. The focus had to be on who the patient was *in the moment*. In this way, the patient became an active participant in the pattern recognition, not just a recipient of custodial care. A primary aspect of the model was unconditional acceptance of the patient as a person. Ruka pointed out that patients with dementia never lose the ability to feel emotions. In the vagueness of pattern recognition with these patients, the nurse may have felt that something was not right but had not known what to do. Some of the staff were unable to tolerate the uncertainty of these situations, but others were able to "hang in there" trusting the process, which ultimately was liberating. This reliance on feelings is a way of knowing that must be cultivated in nursing.

TRANSFORMING PRACTICE

HEC praxis, based as it is on an open-ended, evolving theory, is continuing to evolve in relation to the nature of the clients, the theoretical understanding of the practitioner/researcher, and the particular circumstances. Meaningful directions have started to emerge from the data. The characteristics of higher consciousness have been revealed by research depicting persons facing life-threatening diseases and other crises. Nurses practicing within this perspective experience the joy of participating in the transformation of others and find that their own lives are enhanced and transformed in the process of the dialogue. Once nurses experience the paradigm shift and view patient situations from the standpoint of HEC, it is difficult, if not impossible, for them to view nursing practice any other way. Flanagan (2000) related that both nurses and patients feel "lucky" and "blessed" to have been a part of the experience. Berry (2000) said "HEC has been a strong foundation for . . . my day-to-day practice as a nurse practitioner. . . . The world view allows a connection like no other."

The experiences of these practitioner/researchers convince me that the goal of nursing is to provide a transforming presence for those in need of nursing care. A client shared her perspective:

It was a time of my life in which I was on a treadmill. I just couldn't stop for fear that I would lose all hope of keeping up. I was in a responsible faculty position at a college that was located 90 minutes from my home, so I was involved in a long, stressful daily commute. My husband had accepted a new position across the country; he was working there. Our house was for sale in anticipation of a family move at the end of the academic year. I had three children: one was a teenager getting into some risky behaviors; one a 10-year-old, and a new baby only 3 months old. I had always taken pride in my strength and self-reliance, my ability to be able to do it all! Suddenly, I noticed that I was having a very difficult time picking up the baby. My wrists were very painful at the base of my thumbs. Any movement of my thumbs was excruciating! I called my physician, who told me that it was tendonitis, and that it wasn't uncommon for it to happen after a pregnancy. He said he would treat it by injecting the tendon sheath with cortisone.

I called a friend, a nurse who embodied the unitary perspective. During our conversation, I described my painful hands and how I just couldn't do anything with them because of the pain. She asked me about what was happening in my life, and of course I shared the stress and strain of being alone and responsible for my children and the job, having to keep the house in shape for "showings" and the draining daily commute. I remember the conversation so vividly. I remember it feeling like I was releasing a burden as I told her all this. She paused after I had finished. It was an important silence in which I sensed our close connection. Softly, she said, "Sounds to me like you just can't handle all this by yourself any longer." I started to laugh and cry at the same time . . . I thought, "How profound that my body is giving me this message about my life!" I experienced a feeling of expansion . . . of freedom, like I was soaring! Everything looked brighter somehow. This stunning insight into what was going on with me, this pattern recognition, had set me free. My nurse friend and I continued to talk and I made decisions about getting some additional help with child care and cleaning. We talked about my seeing my self-worth tied to all the many things I could take on and accomplish. I made plans for more rest and time at home. I was on a different path.

Yes, I got my cortisone injection the next day and the pain was relieved. But my nurse addressed the more important issues that helped me to live my life differently. I've never forgotten that conversation with my friend, the nurse. It has been an enduring presence that changed my life.

Nurses who have participated in this process of expanding consciousness have witnessed firsthand the differences in clients' vitality, sense of self, and personal relationships, and in some instances, the healing of their bodies. The nurses report their own transformations as well.

The task in nursing research is to develop knowledge regarding the nurse-patient process in its unity and to recognize the dynamic nature of the evolving process. This process culminates in the intuitive apprehension and expression of the whole system of order of which one is a member. There is a basic way of knowing that is an attunement of the senses, a resonant receptivity. It is intuitive and revelatory and involves senses interacting with environment. This basic way of knowing, *resonance*, necessitates reflective, quiet contemplation. Rogers (1970) established resonancy as an integral process in nursing science:

"Man [sic] experiences his environment as a resonating wave . . . uniting him with the rest of the world. The life process may be likened to cadences—sometimes harmonic, sometimes cacophonous, sometimes dissonant; rising and falling; now fast, now slow—ever changing in a universal orchestration of dynamic wave patterns" (p. 101).

Chapter 4

Resonating with the Whole

Our real identity is consciousness.

Neal Grossman, 2002

. . . in actuality there is only consciousness.

Jose Arguelles, 1987

C onsciousness is the information of the pattern of the whole and is active as well as reflexive (Young, 1976). The essence of the universe is information, and the essence of information is *resonance* (Arguelles, 1987). This information is accessible to us as feeling and meaning. There is nothing without feeling. In attending to feeling, we sense the resonance of incoming information and co-create a resonant field. Schwartz (2006) described this new model of reality:

> All points of consciousness . . . are part of a network of life that they both inform and influence and are informed and influenced by. There is a passage back and forth between the individual and the collective (p. 30).

Before delving into the theoretical aspects of resonancy, I would like to relate an example from nursing practice. By attending to feeling, Capasso (2005) experienced the resonance of the interpenetrating field of her relationship as a clinical nurse specialist with an elderly woman client. The client had slow-healing venous stasis leg ulcers with severe edema and had been referred to Capasso because of difficulties in maintaining consistent contact with medical care professionals. Capasso's intent was to approach the client within the context of the theory of health as expanding consciousness; she was committed to a deep connection with this client. By chance, Capasso's mention of her son's having the flu triggered the woman's memories of the 1918 flu epidemic and that period of her life as one of rejection and disconnection. After about an hour of relating difficulties within her family and with neighbors, the client suddenly displayed deep anguish, revealed a lifelong secret regarding being sexually abused by an adoptive father and began to sob. Capasso, even though feeling uncertain as to what to do, remained fully present and compassionate and expressed total acceptance of the woman's revelation and behavior. When the client had recovered her composure, Capasso proceeded with dressing the wounds and made other suggestions appropriate to the medical care. At the next visit a week later Capasso was astounded to see **marked** reduction in the edema and a 50 percent decrease in the depth of the ulcers. The client's response was: "You know you really helped me last week."

The change in the client's condition could not be explained by treatment regimen or difference in the care of the wounds. What did happen was that Capasso was able to concentrate fully and unconditionally on what was most meaningful to the client, to help her get to the essence of her long-term pattern of isolation and abuse, and allow the breakthrough of insight with the expression of the repressed sorrow. Letting go of the long-held secret was accompanied by a release of tears and the fluid retention in her legs and the freeing of energy for healing. Capasso herself was transformed by this experience in her realization of the power of her presence. She was made vividly aware of coming to know the whole person through the "window of an illness." There was no way to predict what would happen or to know the answers to the problems. One could only be steadfast in being fully present and feeling as one with the client. Figure 4–1 illustrates the coming together of nurse and patient, the resonant pulsating as One in pattern recognition, and the transformation that takes place as they move apart. A similar trajectory may be seen in other instances of praxis in Chapter 3.

Transformation may be explained by the transductive wave properties of all information: that is, the ability to pass directly from one condition of being to another, as when, in an octave, one tone can be sounded to produce its overtones in other octaves. It is communicated by virtue of its pattern of information. "The information that binds all explicated particles together and makes them part of one whole can be termed *nonenergetic* information. All points in space-time have immedi-

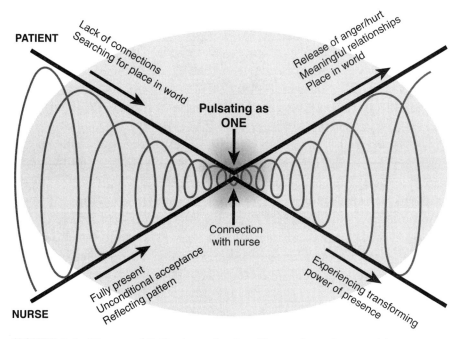

FIGURE 4–1. Nurse and Patient coming together and moving apart in process recognition, insight, and transformation.

ate access to this vast storehouse, since nonenergetic information does not travel through space-time . . . there is no flow of energy" (Friedman, 1990, p. 263, emphasis added). Implicate information is nonenergetic; sensory information, such as heat and touch, is energetic. Lindbergh (1972) added that he suspects that extrasensory and sensory perception will prove to be different faces of each other, as can be seen in the Capasso example.

This is an important distinction in the explication of nursing knowledge. Knowledge at the unitary, transformative level includes and transcends energy transfer at the sensorial level. It is *nonenergetic, nonlocal, and present everywhere*. The cumulative learning effect, which Sheldrake (1983) attributed to morphogenetic fields, supports resonance as the mechanism for learning. The fields are conceived as being without mass or energy, and the effect is not diminished by space or time. This mechanism of information transfer explains the immediacy of transformation by way of resonance.

Meaning is an essential feature of consciousness and is the essence of the implicate order (Friedman, 1990). Meaning can be equated with pattern. It is the common ground of all forms of matter. Taylor, a former cancer researcher/philosopher, equated consciousness and meaning and asserted that evolution is a process of the accumulation of meaning. The human body contains more meaning than any other matter and as such is the highest level of evolution on planet earth. All manifestations are centered in meaning. Motion and time serve to communicate meaning, which transcends changes in matter (Taylor, 1972).

What we call "time" is the simultaneous movement out from and back to the galactic core. As long as we are attuned to time going in only one direction, what we perceive of the galaxy and the universe is only half the picture (Arguelles, 1987). The basic way of knowing is through attunement, resonant receptivity, intuition, revelation—a direct, unfiltered index of communication between the senses and the environment. This involves the capacity to become *selfless* through reflective silence, quiet contemplation, and meditation (Arguelles, 1984).

The whole organizes the parts, and any event happening anywhere is immediately available everywhere as information. ***All wave fronts coming into point X pass on information to X, so that point X contains information from all other points, and vice versa*** (Friedman, 1990). Figure 4–2 is intended to represent this availability of information from all points to the person, and vice versa. This concept is important for the nurse in tapping into the pattern of the whole. Muses referred to res-

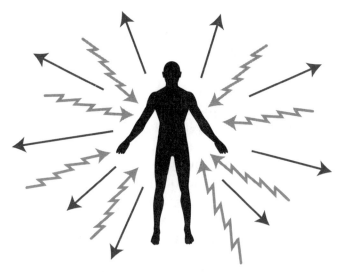

FIGURE 4–2. The Person as the Center of Consciousness with information flow to and from all points in the universe.

onance as radiative causation, a science of resonances that is an all-embracing supersystem of resonances guiding the cosmos. He sees metaphor as the language of meaning, exhibiting clusters that radiate multidimensionally. Again, this analogy rings true for the nurse as he or she senses the pattern of a person in metaphoric terms. Muses rejected the term "acausal" being used to denote phenomena that are nonlineally causal and pointed out that just because lineal causality is insufficient to describe the reality of radiative causation, "the deeper . . . truth is that resonance is simply a higher causal dimension" (Muses, 1985, p. 22).

We can tune into galactic frequencies within our very being (Arguelles, 2002). This basic way of knowing through attunement and resonant receptivity manifests itself in intuition and revelation. Experienced nurses are rife with instances of intuitive insights in the care of their patients. Contrariwise, intellectualization breaks the field of resonance. If we analyze or evaluate an experience before we have resonated with it, the field is broken—the resonance is damped. This loss of resonance explains what happens as the novice nurse tries desperately to intellectualize the insights of her or his experienced colleagues.

Arguelles (1985) suggests creating a mandala to illustrate this process for oneself. The center of the mandala represents the universality of one's center, the point from which all goes forth and to which all returns. Expanding consciousness is *following a path to one's center*. Each moment expands out from the center, its pattern containing the configuration of the universe. The healing power of the mandala pulsates to and from the center of individuation to infinite potential (Refer again to Figure 4–2). This continuous fluctuation is reciprocal in that a change in one person is consistent with a change in others. Arguelles (1985, p. 17) describes acceptance of the nature of the experience:

> From the point of view of the Mandala, there are no "good" or "bad" aspects to situations, much less good or bad experiences: all experiences are equal in the sense that they happen at all. It is the individual's task not to assign ethical definitions to his experiences but to accept them equally, to assimilate them and understand the lesson they hold for him.

The capacity for selflessness has been shown to be important in allowing client/participants to accept their own patterns. The nurse must be able to let go of her or his own personal judgments regarding health behaviors (such as smoking or eating) to clear the field for the underlying pattern to emerge. Endo and her colleagues found that one's own closely held values had to be released in order to form open relationships with clients:

> Differences of family culture or belief system between the family participant and nurse-researcher also influenced the interacting pattern and therefore the rhythm of the evolving pattern. For example, one nurse-researcher had a preconceived image of a middle-aged couple's married life and it took more time to understand their life and to grasp their pattern. Another barrier to relating was the nurse-researcher's difficulty in accepting the father's authoritarianism in the family (Endo, Nitta, et al., 2000, p. 608).

A practicing nurse in another setting shared the importance of letting go of her "ought to" and "should" attitudes based on her religious beliefs in order to eliminate those barriers to an open relationship with her clients (Newman, Lamb, & Michaels, 1991).

How do we reconcile this nondichotomous view of experience with previous allusions to illness as a breakdown or blockage of energy flow (Arguelles, 1987; Bentov, 1977)? Peat (1991) offered an explanation that it is difficult to distinguish between chaos and the flux of ever-changing complexity. Is there a difference, or is the disturbance the chaotic turbulence that precedes reorganization at a higher level? Living systems "are sustained by highly complex fields of cooperative information . . . an ever-flowing, ever-changing pattern of meaning becomes life itself" (Peat, 1991, p. 105). I conclude that the disturbance is an aspect of the ongoing patterning of expanding consciousness, as in the disequilibrium phase of Prigogine's process of dissipative structures. Chaos is enfolded in order and continues at a deeper level with an even deeper order. Chance events reveal the superorder in which all events are embedded (as can be seen in the previous nursing encounter by Capasso). The implication is that there is not a direct lineal causal connection between events, but rather that the relationship takes place in the flux of the holomovement (Friedman, 1990, 1994). This includes disturbances experienced as illness or disruptive events in the ongoing fluctuation of expanding consciousness.

How does the nurse get in touch with this level of order? There is no established procedure for sensing into the whole, but knowing that resonant properties have been documented as characteristic of DNA, and of DNA's response to pulsating fields (Smith, 2006), one can pay attention to the messages of the client at the simplest level. One begins with whatever level presents itself. Assume it is purposeful.

A WAY OF SEEING

The whole indeed is contained in the part.
Jose Arguelles, 1987

It is difficult to fathom the enormity of wholeness. The mode of consciousness associated with logical thinking, so prevalent in the academic world, is necessarily analytical, which is also associated with language. This analytical structure is focused on the level of the word instead of meaning, which is not present in the same linear manner as words. The holistic mode of consciousness is *nonlinear, simultaneous, intuitive, and concerned with relationships rather than the elements that are related.*

This way of seeing cannot be understood by the verbal-intellectual mind, where it is not possible to appreciate adequately what it means to say that a relationship can be experienced as something real in itself. In the analytical mode, the elements stand out rather than the relationship (e.g., sodium and chlorine rather than the bond that makes them salt). The experience of a relationship requires a transformation from piecemeal thought to simultaneous perception of the whole. The experience of simultaneity and relationship in the holistic mode of consciousness is inherently dynamical.

Bortoft's (1986, 1996) explication of Goethe's way of seeing is helpful. Rather than focusing on lineal causal order, as in mainstream science, Goethe focused on seeing the whole. At the same time he pointed out that the whole is present *in* the parts and can be encountered through the parts. To be clear, the whole is not made up of parts but is *reflected* in the parts. He gave the example of the whole expanse of sky being present in light, which interacts with the pupil of the eye: "here is everywhere and everywhere is here" (1996, p. 5). The old scientific view of the universe as matter made up of separate masses is replaced by the view that mass is not an intrinsic property of a body, but a reflection of the whole of the universe in that body. One cannot perceive the whole by "standing back to get an overview" but by going further into the parts (p. 6)—by going further into the center of self and seeing the phenomenon anew.

In referring to hermeneutics, Bortoft (1996) reminded us that reading is an act of interpretation (not just a matter of saying words) that conveys *meaning*, which relates to the whole text: ". . . the meaning of the text is discerned . . . with progressive immanence . . ." (p. 7). The meaning is analogous to the whole picture in a hologram: "The whole is present throughout all of the text, so that it is present in any part of the text" (p. 8). There is the paradox of needing to understand authors before we read their works and yet having to read their works first in order to understand. ". . . it is the *experience* we go through to understand the meaning . . ." (Bortoft, p. 8). Listeners also bring their own context to the meaning of what is read. Sometimes the understanding of a single passage suddenly illuminates the whole meaning. This occurrence is particularly relevant in nursing practice when one word or phrase that the client utters, sometimes rather inadvertently, captures the wholeness of the situation. To the sensitive nurse, this breakthrough is an "aha" moment.

Much of our educational experience involves logic. Logic is analytical and leads away from grasping the whole. Meaning is holistic. "We understand meaning in the moment of *coalescence* when the whole is reflected in the parts so that together they disclose the whole" (Bortoft, 1996, p. 9). The conventional way of knowing is summative and integrative, with the implication that the whole comes later than the parts. What we need to understand is the *primacy* of the whole, echoing Bohm's (1980) position that wholeness is what is real, with fragmentation as our response to fragmentary thought. The whole is irreducible and omnipresent. "Thus the whole emerges simultaneously with the accumulation of the parts, not because it is the sum of the parts, but because it is immanent within them" (Bortoft, 1996, p. 9).

The part is a place for *being present with the whole*. When the whole of a phenomenon seems overwhelming and the task of studying it impossible, it is comforting to know we can enter into the whole through the parts, which may look different without the vision of the whole. To return to an example from Pharris' (2002; 2005) study, an adolescent's commitment of murder looks different when viewed in isolation than it does when the total pattern of his life, family, and community are considered. The overall pattern of participants in Pharris' study depicted highly interactive youths experiencing blocked relationships with their parents during their early childhood. They described the aloneness of having absentee fathers and mothers addicted to alcohol or other drugs. Frequent moves accentuated their sense of isolation. They each experienced at least one critical event of assault or separation that accentuated their sense of isolation and appeared to precipitate a change in their life pattern. They began getting in trouble at school and in the community and were sent to juvenile detention at least once. They began losing their connection to school and felt that the teachers and other officials did not want them there. Most stopped going to school regularly at about age 13. They sought community connections, which turned out to be gangs or other boys involved in delinquent behaviors. They spoke of yearning for positive maternal attention. Before the murder, they all were using marijuana and alcohol on a regular basis. They began carrying guns in order to survive in frequent shootouts, or for robbery. Feelings of anxiety and depression began to break through despite heavy drug use. The feeling that life had no value had a suicidal component as they aimed at and were aimed at by other young men just like themselves. The murders were committed in a haze of distorted time, movement, and space. As one young man described it, it was like being in slow motion in a movie. Being in prison gave them an opportunity to slow down and look within. It was at that time that Pharris began meeting with them to discuss what was meaningful to them.

The patterns of the individuals reflected a reciprocal community pattern: The trajectory of the life patterns of these young men portrayed a lack of nurturance in the home, disconnection with the school and legitimate community organizations, and availability of the street drug industry. Cut off from positive interaction with their family, school, and noncriminal community organizations, the whole could be seen in the isolated, alienated parts. When this community pattern was shared with community agencies and groups, they recognized the points of disconnection and gained insight regarding their opportunities for action to reconnect with the alienated youth (Pharris, 2005).

The whole is encountered by stepping right into the parts. There is a dual movement of moving through the parts to enter into the whole. If we do not understand this, we merely pass along the parts without seeing the whole. Endo (personal communication, 2006), for example, shared her experience of relating to students who wanted to quit smoking. The idea was to use the perspective of health as expanding consciousness (HEC) as the context for a participative study with these students. Her expectation was, not that they would quit smoking within this context, but that they would experience some changes in their lives through recognition of their own patterns. She was willing to approach the students from the standpoint of pattern recognition of the whole. In the student-teacher partnerships that were formed within HEC, the students did indeed recognize their patterns and new patterns evolved: new relationships with their parents, new relationships with their friends, new eating and study patterns. They did not quit smoking right away, but made plans to do so and later sent e-mails back to the faculty researchers reporting that even some of the heavy smokers had eliminated smoking from their new life pattern. The focus here was on pattern of the whole, but from the participants' standpoint initially the entry was based on a particular behavior.

We need to be alert to what Bortoft (1996) referred to as "spectator awareness:" In the moment of recognizing a thing, we stand outside of that thing ". . . and turn into an 'I' . . ." (pp. 13–14). We become an observer, and the observed becomes a thing. This way of seeing was a factor in the reporting of some of the early studies of pattern recognition (Newman & Moch, 1991; Newman, 1995). It appeared as though we were standing outside the client and describing the pattern of a "thing." In reality we were engaged in a caring presence with the client in the mutual process of exploring the meaning of their lives as it evolved. The transformative power of the dialogue was active even though our written descriptions of the patterning failed to communicate its presence. We were engaged in the articulation of wholeness through compassionate consciousness (Skolimowski, 1994).

Bortoft (1996) spoke of the whole as an active absence, such as occurs in the enacting of a play. The actors "enter into a part in such a way that they enter into the play. But actors do not encounter the play as an object of knowledge over which they can stand like the lines they learn. They encounter the play in their part as an active absence which can begin to move them. . . . an actor starts to be acted by the play . . . the play speaks through them," (p. 15) and they interact with each other. From my experience as an author, the author begins to be guided by the book. So we encounter the whole, not as an object but as an active absence. In this way, we understand that in the nurse-client dialogue, it is not the words of the dialogue that matter, but the active, unseen pattern of the process. At the same time that we recognize that the whole is not a thing, we know that it is not mere nothing, but it is invisible to the scientific approach as currently conceived. Silva, Sorrell, and Sorrell (1995) acknowledged this kind of knowledge of the "in-between" and "beyond" as important to nursing.

Goethe (Bortoft, 1986) proposed a radically different way of doing science. What was important to Goethe was the *process*, the *perspective*, not the factual content about the object of study (p. 8). Goethe's approach avoided reducing the phenomenon and rather finding the wholeness by perceiving the relationships as they present themselves. His important contribution to science was his way of seeing, a way of seeing that cannot be grasped like an object. It is the "unity of the world" (p. 9). Unity is not locatable in space-time (e.g., like contrast: one can see a black bowl on a white table, but the contrast between them is not locatable). To understand Goethe's way of seeing we have to experience it for ourselves. We can only really understand it by participation. This necessity provides an important reminder for nursing education: In order to learn this way of seeing, one must have an opportunity to experience it.

One way to accomplish this is by involving students in the experience of pattern recognition. Endo (personal communication, 2006) pointed out that in her study with students who wanted to quit smoking, the students were involved in a more active role in the partnership process. They listened to the tape recording of each dialogue session with the faculty member and made a summary of their life pattern with notes about any added new awareness they experienced. The faculty/researcher did the same, and at the beginning of the next session they shared each other's perception of the evolving pattern. In this way, the students were learning to experience the evolving process, a learning that they could utilize in assisting patients.

The unity of a phenomenon is experienced in the present rather than the past and is an event in which we learn to participate. It is not repeatable, a factor that has implications for research. Goethe's way of seeing is experienced uniquely in each participant situation. We must learn to *receive the presence* of the other person.

A SENSE OF UNITY

The world that we experience is not visible to the somatic senses. There is an extra, nonsensory, factor that transforms sensory experience. Bortoft (1986) illustrated the extra factor with the familiar drawing of a duck-rabbit (Fig. 4–3). What you see (a duck or a rabbit) is a function of an organizing factor of perception; it is not in the actual sensory input.

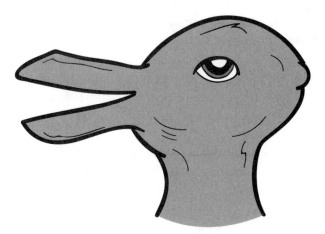

FIGURE 4–3. Duck/rabbit drawing.

The wholeness that we see **is** the meaning, not the meaning **of** what is seen, but the meaning which **is** what is seen. What we are seeing is not in fact on the page, even though it appears to be there. The mind organizes experience by *imposing* an organizational framework. When we see a "chair," we have already attached meaning to what we see.

Paradoxically: "But the unity which Goethe perceived in the . . . phenomenon is *not* a unity that is imposed by the mind. What Goethe saw was not an intellectual unification but the wholeness of the phenomenon itself. He came to see the wholeness of the phenomenon by . . . experiencing it, and this experience cannot be reduced to an intellectual construction . . . It is not reached by a process of intellectual thought, but by a change of consciousness . . ." (Bortoft, 1986, p. 27). The unity that is perceived in this way **is** the phenomenon—but not the phenomenon as it is immediately accessible to the senses. This unity is an experience of seeing the phenomenon in depth; there is no intellectual equivalent to this experience. The intuitive experience of seeing this unity **is** the theory for Goethe. The method is the theory. This also is true for nursing: the way of seeing the pattern of the whole **is** the theory of nursing.

Goethe's sense of unity without unification is within the phenomenon itself, not an intellectual unity of unification. Unity without unification is the unity of the intuitive mind. "The unity 'lights up' in consciousness—it is insight . . . The phenomenon is only partially visible to the senses. The complete phenomenon is visible only when there is a coalescence of sensory outsight and noetic insight" (Bortoft, 1986, p. 29).

Goethe's way of knowing is intuitive, the roots of which means "seeing into." It is the experience of seeing the phenomenon in depth. "This intensive depth which is seen intuitively in the holistic mode of consciousness **is** the wholeness of the phenomenon" (p. 35). The authentic unity of the phenomenon is literally a further dimension of the phenomenon itself. The intellectual mind misses this dimension. To repeat, if we intellectualize an experience before we have resonated with it, the field is broken; the resonance is damped. For instance, sometimes when we see familiar symptoms of a disease, we jump to a diagnostic conclusion and preclude receptivity to other data that would present a more complete picture. It assumes that we are all the same.

Bortoft (1996, p. 128) cautioned that "where our thinking usually begins, it is already too late. We have to go to the stage prior to our usual awareness . . ." We must engage in a participant mode of consciousness rather than an onlooker mode. When one comes to a choice point and conceives of an action, that **is** action.

To return to a previous illustration, seeing a chair is a way of seeing, but is not pure sensory perception, which takes away all conceptualization (Bortoft, 1996). Before seeing a chair, one must have a concept of a chair. Our experience is the coalescence of an organizing idea (a chair) with the sensory information. In the duck/rabbit figure (see Fig. 3), each picture is wholly the figure (not part of it), and yet no one picture exhausts the figure. Meaning **is** what we see. Our theoretical persuasion structures what we see. If we're looking for pathology, we see pathology; if we're looking for pattern, we see pattern.

What is lost in strict empiricism is the active role of the theory. This loss may be seen in the emphasis on scientific evidence-based practice; the evidence may be an instrumental relationship without a nursing theoretical base. Transformation in what we see is a function of our way of seeing, our theoretical perspective. The visual appearance remains the same, but the meaning is different. If the organizing idea changes, then what is seen changes. When I was exploring the nature of nursing practice of a group of case managers, I was alert to instances in their practice of pattern recognition and assistance to clients at choice points in their lives; what I saw was a function of my theory, the organizing idea of health as expanding consciousness (HEC). Had I been looking through the lens of another framework, say caring, that would have influenced what I saw (Newman, Lamb, and Michaels, 1991). The link between theory and what is seen makes an important difference in practice.

Goethe's way of seeing is imaginal rather than material. This requires a highly evolved individual and has implications for the education necessary for this capacity to develop. We need to develop the quality of seeing comprehensively rather than selectively. It is clear that a change in the way of seeing transforms what is seen without changing the content. "When things are seen in context, so that intrinsic connections are revealed, then the experience we have is that of *understanding*," (Bortoft, 1996, p. 290) which is not the same as explaining, which replaces one thing with another. Explaining is reductionistic, analytical. The need is to see connections directly (wholeness) with nothing new added. Understanding reveals the phenomenon fully as itself. In this way, we experience both kinds of seeing together—seeing in different ways simultaneously. When we recognize a chair, we see the physical attributes (sensory input) and recognize them as fitting the category of a "chair" (imaginal seeing) at the same time.

Activities of analysis and synthesis are a step removed from the living present of the process to the dead past of the product. To avoid this pitfall, we need to shift from what is seen to the *seeing* quality itself. The key factor is the organizing idea, the theory. To illustrate, Bortoft (1996) suggested picturing a giraffe embedded in black and white blotches (Fig. 4–4). The markings on the page are the same; what is different is the *seeing experience*. Contrary to empiricism, the giraffe is in the seeing, not on the page. The way of seeing and what is seen cannot be separated. This dynamic approach seeks to catch the process instead of starting from the finished product. As Bortoft suggested, seeing the giraffe is seeing "giraffely." In nursing, seeing the pattern is seeing "patternly." This is an important learning task for students of nursing.

Goethe's sense of unity is experienced as a way of seeing that includes differences, avoids reducing multiplicity to uniformity, and avoids fragmenting reality. "It allows the uniqueness of the particular to appear within the light of the unity of the whole" (Bortoft, 1996, p. 248). Wholeness is a higher dimension of the phenomenon and is not to be confused with seeing generally; it is the capacity to comprehend differences as a unity. This way of seeing allows the uniqueness of each pattern to emerge. The higher level is the experience of meaning (pattern); that is, when we *see* the connection rather than *introducing* one. Goethe (Bortoft, 1996) detested the "craving for generality" (p. 301), which he saw as the preoccupation of science. Seeing comprehensively is concrete

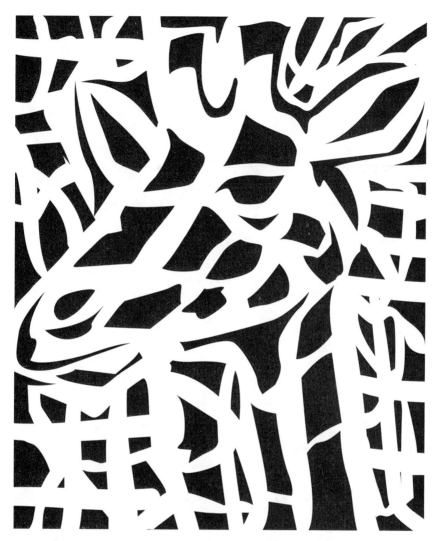

FIGURE 4–4. Giraffe embedded in black and white blotches.

and holistic, whereas generalization is abstract and analytical; these ways of seeing go in opposite directions.

These different ways of seeing explain the difference between general and universal (Bortoft, 1986, p. 49). The general is an abstraction based on many particulars. It is counterfeit for universal and is arrived at by the intellectual, analytical mind. The universal is the One (one which is many) and is experienced by the intuitive, holistic mind. In intellectual consciousness one moves from particulars to general—an abstraction. For the intuitive mind, there is reversal of perception: there is perception of the universal in the particular, which is a concrete manifestation of the universal. The particular becomes symbolic of the universal. "So what is merely particular to the senses . . . is simultaneously universal to an intuitive way of seeing which is associated with a different mode of consciousness" (Bortoft, 1986, p. 43). Goethe saw the intuitive unity of a plant: that all forms are metamorphic variations of one form, reflecting the principle that the whole is reflected in the part. The leaf is "an instance worth a thousand, bearing all within itself" (Bortoft, 1986, p. 45).

Nevertheless, generalization does occur, as in the synthesized pattern derived from patterns of individuals in most of the HEC studies, which yields a kind of unity in multiplicity in which difference is excluded (from the many to the one). This abstraction may be helpful as a prospective tool, as in Pharris' projection of the pattern of community from the pattern of individuals and in the development of models of practice. Nursing practitioners should be aware, though, of Bortoft's (1996) caution:

> We tend toward generalizing by abstraction whenever we begin with the finished product instead of with the process of coming-into-being. In this case we confront the finished product—the set of chairs—as an onlooker: there is a set of different objects, and what they have in common is that each one is a chair. So the process of generalization takes the form of finding unity in multiplicity, identity in diversity. The unity is abstracted from the multiplicity, drawn off it externally by standing back from the multiplicity as an onlooker to find what is common. In seeking for what is common in this way, all difference is excluded. Hence there can be no diversity within unity when unity is understood this way, and all that remains is uniformity (p. 249).

Like many of us, Goethe had to emancipate himself from the idol of empiricism. He saw inductive generalization as *lifeless*. Lifeless observations contribute little to an understanding of the uniqueness of individuals in process. Goethe developed a way of looking for an instance indicative of the whole. Whereas intellectually we see many in the form of one, intuitively we see One (the universal) in the form of many. (I felt this kind of intuitive sense of the whole in regard to my mother's illness experience.) "Hence each of the many is the very same One" (Bortoft, 1986, p. 50) in a way that *includes* difference instead of eradicating it. It is important in nursing to concentrate on the One, the universality of each encounter, and at the same time to honor the diversity. We need to include this way of knowing in the nursing curriculum.

The key to Goethe's way of seeing is the unity of wholeness:

> . . . failure to see how the many are One leads us to try to produce some kind of synthesis of the many, i.e., to make One from one. But the "One" which we try to reach from the many can only be the counterfeit made by an external synthesis of many ones or the abstract uniformity of what many ones have in common. The One is the many—we could say it is "hidden" in the many, hidden by our customary way of seeing" (Bortoft, 1996, p. 257).

A bamboo plant, for instance, appears to be many separate plants, but it propagates itself by producing new shoots underground. An entire forest is One plant (One in the form of many). The whole is present within its parts, but never coming into presence totally and finally in any one part. When we seek to find what is common to the many, we achieve an abstraction, which moves "away from the authentic unity of living wholeness to the counterfeit unity of abstract uniformity" (Bortoft, 1996, p. 261).

The many plants that are one (generalization, abstraction) and the One plant which is many (universal, holistic) are really different dimensions of the same phenomenon. Similarly a pattern may manifest itself in many forms. The method of "active looking" followed by exact sensorial imagination is the key. This promotes the holistic mode. Compared with observable parts, the pattern of the organism as a whole seems to be nebulous and unreal. It seems as if it belongs more to the mind of the beholder than to the organism itself. Nevertheless, Goethe was sure that the pattern of the organism was something real and not just a figment in the mind of the beholder. Actually, in a worldview in which there is no separation of observer and observed, the experience is co-created. It is intuitive knowledge gained through contemplation: the exercise of thinking inwardly as well as outwardly, the exercise of trying to see the visible aspect as a whole—experiencing the phenomenon intuitively as well as sensorially. I am reminded of my original intuition that all manifestations of the person reflect the underlying pattern, that disease is a manifestation of the whole, and later, that the observable patterns of relating reflect physical patterns of exchange. It is not a matter of collecting data from many individuals to portray the whole but of intuiting the whole from the pattern of one. The experience of wholeness as a real quality is possible in the holistic, unitary mode of consciousness. In the beginning of our learning to grasp the whole, we may flip back and forth between the intellectual and the intuitive, between the sensorial and the meaning, but we can be assured that they are all dimensions of the whole.

Our ability to know things is integral with where we are in the evolving process. Expanding consciousness is integral to the evolution of all that there is, and we can know only from that perspective (Kremer, 1992). A practitioner in HEC testified to the importance of his own level of consciousness in resonating with the realm of consciousness of the nurse-client process:

> It was a personal and professional stretch to look at the whole, to deal with areas I hadn't dealt with before . . . As one grows professionally and personally, new options open up. I'm sharing my experience with the person, [just] as what they're going through is offered to me. I hear things and recognize things in people that I wouldn't have before, might have dealt with differently (Newman, Lamb, and Michaels, 1991, pp. 406–407).

Goethe saw knowledge of a phenomenon as being intimately related to the phenomenon itself. For him the state *of being known* was understood as *a further stage* of the phenomenon itself. Consequently the knower is not an onlooker but a participant in nature's processes, which act to reveal the unfolding pattern. Goethe remarked that the aim of science should be that "through the contemplation of an ever creating nature, we . . . make ourselves worthy of spiritual participation in her production" (Bortoft, 1986, p. 66). He saw "being known" as a higher stage of the phenomenon, which is not complete without it. The significance of intuitive knowledge is manifest in this process in which the phenomenon itself comes into presence: "The act of knowing is an evolutionary development of the phenomenon . . ." (Bortoft, 1986, p. 66). In this way, the nurse-patient mutual process becomes the instrument by which nurses and patients move to a higher stage of themselves. A person's potential is recognized as others come to know it and become part of it.

Chapter 5

Being Fully Present

Being intensely engaged in relationship with another is one of the greatest joys of being human. It is, perhaps, the most vital manifestation of consciousness. . . . This approach to consciousness calls for a shift of perspective–from looking at the world as a collection of objects, or even as a collection of subjects, to a view which sees relationship as fundamental.

Christian de Quincey, 2005

Viewing relationship as fundamental to the study of consciousness emphasizes its importance in the development of nursing knowledge. The relationship between the nurse and the client has been referred to as "the essence of nursing" (The American Nurse, Sept-Oct 1998). For the discipline, the emphasis on relationship means that knowledge development focuses on process as content.

The essence of the process is in being fully present in the transformation of ourselves and others as we search for meaning in the lives of persons who have come to critical junctures in their lives. Many persons with coronary heart disease, for instance, are faced with the aloneness of their previous aggressive lifestyle and the need to develop more meaningful relationships (Newman & Moch, 1991). The diagnosis of cancer brings with it an important turning point (LeShan, 1989) and highlights the need for attention to quality of life and relationships (Barron, 2005; Endo, 1998; Kiser-Larson, 2002; Moch, 1990; Newman, 1995a). Persons living with the AIDS virus are confronted with the need to find balance in their interaction with the environment and in the nature of their relationships (Lamendola & Newman, 1994). Persons with dementia are particularly sensitive to the presence of others in their environment but often are unable to express their sense of relatedness or may express this relatedness in an unfamiliar way (Ruka, 2005).

Whereas the task of medicine is to counteract the disease process, the mission of nursing is to help the client find meaning in the evolving process. The nature of nursing practice is the caring, pattern-recognizing relationship between nurse and client—a relationship that is a transforming presence.

Rogers (1970) identified mutual process as an essential dimension of her revolutionary ideas about unitary nature. She set the stage for the development of nursing knowledge on the basis of relationship, replacing the notion of separate parts interacting with that of dynamic, simultaneous, changing relations. Relating with another occurs as trust is established and authenticity recognized. The ability of the nurse and patient to relate and connect with the other in a meaningful way occurs in dialogue. Meaning unfolds within the dialogical process of nurse and patient. As insight occurs, action potential is apparent.

Spradlin and Porterfield (1984) were adamant regarding the importance of relationship. In their study of patterns and relationships, rather than actions of entities: "One cannot separate individual consciousness from the web of an event. . . . The self is, then, the area of a pulsating circle . . . [and] has no meaning without reference points in a relationship. There is no self without relationship" (pp. 232, 234). Bateson (1979) emphasized relationship thinking and, consistent with his focus on the pattern that connects, suggested that relationship be used as a basis for all definition. Capra (1982) added that Bateson believed that anything should be defined not only by what it is, but by its relations to others.

According to deQuincey (1998), Buber regarded Feuerbach's insight—that is, the essence of human being as *relationship*—as comparable to the Copernican revolution. De Quincey further claimed that the essence of the human being is found in community, in the unity of person and person. He suggested that a crucial aspect of the "new" paradigm may be the awareness of our deep intersubjective nature and concluded that the ideal of intersubjective knowledge is relationship: "There is something about the nature of consciousness . . . that requires the *presence* of the 'other' as another subject which can acknowledge my being. (When I experience myself being experienced by you, my experience of myself—and

you—is profoundly enriched, even, in some encounters, 'transformed')"
(p. 46). Even at the subatomic level, the atom exists as a *set of relationships.* The in-betweenness of presence is seen as a mysterious force that
represents a fundamental reality of mutuality.

PRESENCE

*. . . authentic presence between patient and nurse. . .
[is] a transformation of both. Presence is a matter of
consciousness and is reflected in the holistic beings that
are both nurses and patients.*

Susan K. Chase, 2001

Being fully present is essential to a transforming relationship. The concept of presence evokes a variety of meaning. It has been described as
genuine dialogue, commitment, full engagement and openness, the core
element of nursing activity, free-flowing attentiveness, transcendent to-
getherness, and transcendent oneness (Smith, 2001). Smith suggested
that when the nurse considers the patient a "mystery" to be engaged in
rather than a "problem" to be solved, the relationship is characterized by
presence. Presence is enhanced by the nurse's openness and sensitivity
to the other.

Doona, Chase, and Haggerty (1999) summed up their findings regarding presence as demonstrating the uniqueness of both the client
and the nurse, connectedness with the client's experience, sensing of
the present moment, going beyond scientific data, **knowing** what will
work and when to act, and the sine qua non: **being with** the client.
Miller and Douglas (1998) agreed that presence involves putting everything else aside and focusing completely on the client; that is, being
with the individual with all aspects of oneself. They saw it as an invita-
tion "to see, to share, to touch, and to hear the vulnerability and suffering of another" (p. 29).

Melnechenko (2003) described Rosemarie Parse's concept of true
presence as a way of being that values the other's dignity and freedom to
choose and is more than caring or active listening. Melnechenko concluded that "true presence creates the opportunity for nurses to go

where the patient is in life, to learn about the experience of health as it is defined and lived, and to work with patients as they choose the meaning of the situation" (p. 23). This intent is consistent with that of nurses practicing within the context of health as expanding consciousness.

As previously noted, consciousness pervades all things (Bentov, 1977; de Quincey, 2005; Gilbert, 2006; Muses, 1978). According to de Quincey, the way of knowing all levels of consciousness is by "a form of non-sensory, non-linguistic connection through *presence* and *meaning,* rather than through mechanism or exchange of energy" (p. 2, emphasis added). Thus any comprehensive investigation of consciousness must include an *engaged presence* of being-in-relationship (p. 27). There is also a sense of purposefulness in this type of relationship.

Presence is a nonsensory prehension of the being of the "other"— the felt enfolding of the "other's" being into a unity that transcends the dichotomy of separate subject and object (deQuincey, 2005, p. 175). As an epistemology of presence, process-oriented intersubjectivity focuses on a deep exploration of relationship. The emphasis is on engagement rather than measurement, on meaning rather than mechanism.

Engaged presence includes and transcends reason and somatic feeling. Words and ideas facilitate instrumental knowing but separate us from intuitive knowing (de Quincey, 2005). Our educational background orients us to the "truth" of propositions but blocks the wisdom of experiential, intuitive knowing. In contrast, recall the maxim of Jose Arguelles, that we should "stand in the center" of our truth. That truth does not exist just for ourselves as individuals but is the essence of our relationships with all things at all times. **It is essential to being fully present.** "Truth" is not just the gathering of facts; it is a relationship between the knowing subject and the rest of the unfolding universe (de Quincey, 2005). It involves a vulnerability in the openness needed to find truth.

So the world is made of processes, of events, rather than entities (things), and the connections are through meaning (pattern) not located in space. The action of our practice, then, is a letting go and becoming one with the resonance of the universe. DeQuincey emphasizes that consciousness does not work like a machine. He makes the case "that when two or more sentient beings engage each other's presence, they know and experience each other mutually through **direct, unmediated, subject-to-subject communion . . .**" (de Quincey, 2005, p. 92, emphasis added).

There is a kind of knowing beyond intuition that is experiential, a kind of "no-knowledge" that transcends all ideas. One must put aside the objects of rational thought and rely on one's awareness of the ineffable. "No-knowledge is a form of knowing where the knower merges with, or participates with, what is known" (deQuincey, 2005, p. 146). This seems to be what is happening when one feels as ONE with another person. From de Quincey: No-knowledge implies "that knowing and being can blend into a single activity: tuning into the consciousness of the object, literally becoming it by experiencing its experience" (p. 150). (Recall Capasso's sensitivity to her client's anguish in Chapter 4.)

In the nurse-patient relationship the focus should be on the connection between the two. We are drawn to look at the nurse or patient because they are concrete entities, and we tend to keep them separate by standing outside and viewing. We need to view the relationship from within and recognize the shared consciousness that occurs. As the nurse is fully present with the patient, the meeting forms a new rhythmic pattern of the combined fields. The nurse "hangs in there" and waits for insight to occur. When it does, the nurse can move away and allow the patient to center in the resonating process without the physical presence of the nurse. The pattern of their transformation persists even though they have moved apart.

No-knowledge brings us to nonaction (in contrast to actions aimed at providing a solution to a problem or treating a malady). This means action not as a means to an end, but as its own reward. It is spontaneous and lets things be. Many people make the present moment into a means to an end, but we never experience the future or the past—only the present moment (Donoso, 2003). Reality is in the present. When one looks to the future, one moves away from the present experience. Being fully present in the experience of the present is the crux of unity consciousness and is essential to nursing practice/research. Even though a nurse may apply knowledge from another discipline to alleviate a problem, the overall perspective is one of past-present-future being fully present in the moment.

Donoso (2003) cites Eckhart Tolle as encouraging a walk in nature with a mind that has become quiet—simply alert presence—pointing to consciousness that is nonconceptual. This relaxed alertness makes it possible for the true presence of being with another to occur. The present— this moment now—is the source of all reality. My experience recently with a woman who has a form of dementia emphasized that for her there is no past or future, only the present. Caregivers need to be aware of the need to be fully present in the present.

What is involved in transforming presence is becoming **one with the client.** This involves letting go of external time and the constraints it imposes on nursing tasks. One must let go and be fully present in the moment. Previously I have stated that consciousness is the informational capacity of the system, and we have sought to identify the evolving pattern of that information. Uncovering patterns has been helpful in understanding the client's situation and in helping the client to gain insights regarding his or her action potential. But becoming one with the client goes beyond pattern identification and is evidence of the unitary transformation taking place.

Falkenstern (2003) described this feeling of oneness with clients as one of timelessness. In her study of the process of the nurse-client relationship with families who had a child with special health-care needs, she deliberately set aside all other commitments and totally focused on the family and their concerns. As she was able to relax into the process of relating to clients, she and the family-client connected rhythmically and timelessly, allowing insights to arise. She recalled, "One does not practice nursing *using* this theory [health as expanding consciousness]. One embodies the theory; the theory becomes a 'way of being' in presencing with the client"(p. 213). She concluded that this experience of oneness and transformation is crucial to the nurse-client relationship in the exploration of potential change. The nurse-client dialogue gives the family an opportunity to tap into the implicate order.

In this paradigm of interconnectedness in which relationship comes first, each of us is a center of the vast network surrounding us, a node in the complex web of life. In this way, each of us is the center of convergence of the resonant field (Refer again to Figure 4–2). One person can know another by engaging her or his presence. Participating in storytelling is a way to evoke meaning because it engages both the storyteller and the listener in shared, common experiences. It is possible to come to know another without words—someone, perhaps, who cannot speak: ". . . one can reach all creatures by a direct connection, consciousness to consciousness, without having to reach the person or creature through his or its body and by means of the senses" (Khan, 1978, p. 12). Pharris (personal communication) shared, "I was keenly aware that I can come to know another without words—that I can resonate with and come to know someone who cannot speak. I need to start with my intention to begin with what is important to the person. If someone can speak, then storytelling centered on what is meaningful is helpful. Somehow that beginning piece of honoring what is important to the person, rather than coming in with a preconceived notion of what is going to happen or be done needs to be emphasized."

Expansion of consciousness is seen as deepening of meaning: Endo (1998), based on her experience of caring for persons with cancer, asserted that expanding consciousness is the accumulation of meaning and that any striving at any stage is an important learning opportunity to develop a higher level of consciousness. Practicing nurses learned "that meaning in nursing situations was not *out there,* but was created in the client-nurse relationship as it was unfolding" (Endo, Suzuki, and Ohmasa, 2005, p. 114). This experience reinforced Endo's earlier assertion of this process as a meaning-making-transformative process.

DeQuincey (2005) refers to sequential events as the passing on of meaning. The body is an information processor, but more than that, a *meaning processor.* According to deQuincey, the *feeling* body is:

- Constantly exchanging information and meaning with the environment.
- Sensitive to messages from the environment.
- A discourse of meaning in dialogue with the world (p. 159).

This process has been called emotional resonance, which connects all sentient beings (Kohanov, 2003) .

The transforming presence that is nursing practice and research has been viewed as a partnership (Jonsdottir, Litchfield, and Pharris, 2003): "The nurse's presence is a fully open caring attentiveness to whatever emerges in the nurse-client relationship. . . . Possibilities for action surface through this unfolding dialogue between nurse and client. They are not solicited or prearranged by the nurse, but emerge as each person uniquely contributes to the dialogue" (pp. 54–55). The partnership ends when the projected actions are explicated retrospectively, indicating how each will move on. Pharris related an example from her practice in which she, as a nurse who was experienced and knowledgeable about recovery from sexual abuse, approached with unconditional acceptance a client who had been sexually abused and assisted her in focusing on the meaning of the experience:

"... I was able to offer her a variety of supportive referrals to choose from. However, what she expressed as being most important was having someone to talk with who obviously cared and who had no ulterior motives or prescribed expectations of what she *should* do. I concentrated on listening to her and to fully attending to what she presented as meaningful to her" (p. 58).

The partnership lasted several months. At termination, the client had gained insight about the experience, recognition of her strengths, and how she had been isolated from the community around her. She had begun making changes to connect with her community. This example illustrates the availability of the nurse with information that can be shared to advance the moment.

Litchfield, too, shared a summary of her partnership with a young mother with five small children, one of whom had experienced multiple, chronic medical diagnoses with repeated exacerbations. It was clear that the episodic care by traditional medical care facilities was unable to address the totality of the situation. Through her interaction with the family over a period of seven visits, they were able to grasp the meaning of the overall pattern of the family's relationships and to gain insight regarding actions to be taken, with the mother seeing her way clear to take charge of her everyday activities with increased vitality. Litchfield learned a year later that the mother's intended actions had been pursued and that "the predicament that had been so devastating and immobilizing had become a fleeting moment in life's trajectory" (p. 59). She concluded that the significance of the partnership continued to unfold over time.

Jonsdottir described an engagement with a couple facing challenges related to the wife's breathing difficulties. The interpersonal conflicts among family members were so intense and the problems so extensive that the nurse doubted her ability to make a difference, but she was committed to staying with the client with the intent to understand the flow of the dialogue and clarify as needed. By the fourth visit a major change had occurred in the interpersonal relationship of the couple and in their relationships with their children. They had made plans to stop smoking and demonstrated a willingness to incorporate the disease condition in their way of life. It became apparent that **knowing** what to do (as a nurse) was transcended by **being fully present.** The process opened the family to the experience. As they became aware of what was happening, they were able to choose. This does not negate the specialized knowledge that the nurse brings to the partnership but illustrates its secondary nature to the unitary, transformative presence of the implicate order. ". . . it is when actions bring coherence to the whole of patients' lives that the transformative nature of changes is revealed . . ." (Jonsdottir, Litchfield, and Pharris, 2004, p. 4).

TRANSCENDING RELATIONSHIPS

Nurses who thrive in relationship with clients in hospice and other situations of terminal care reveal the *sacredness of the ordinary* and the *timelessness of the present* in their work (Lamendola, 1998). Rather than being "burned out" by the strenuous demands of this work, these nurses related how they were nourished and rewarded by their relationships with the patients. A complete elaboration of Lamendola's research was cut short by his untimely death, but his beginning summary gives a glimpse of the essence of his findings:

> The nurse participates with the client in interpenetrating energy fields and expanding consciousness. Both are changed in the relational nature of nursing. The nurse helps through his or her being that goes beyond the doing of tasks that need to be accomplished.
>
> This research began by exploring the possibility that pattern would become apparent for nurses who enjoyed and thrived in their hospice or HIV/AIDS work. What emerged during data analysis was a portrayal of the dimensions of the nursing relationship, dimensions that help to illuminate the theory of nursing based on a concept of health as expanding consciousness. These dimensions are identified as: relatedness, presence, timelessness, ordinariness, and sacredness.
>
> **Relatedness.** Partnership was expressed by the nurses as mutuality and interconnectedness in the nurse-client relationships. The relational nature of nursing practice was very apparent in each nurse's story.
>
> **Presence.** Presence was seen as a "feeling with the other" through listening and physical touch. There was an ease and comfort with the rhythm of their clients in their dying. Presence was also seen as expressions of compassion: being with others in their suffering.
>
> **Timelessness.** Closely tied to presence was a timelessness when the nurse was with a client. The nurse's being in the temporal present and being in the moment with each client was evident, as if there were no distractions—only a sense of being.
>
> **Ordinariness.** The work had a quality of ordinariness to it: Routine and mundane activities repeated over and over again. Yet there was a paradoxical experience of extraordinariness that arose from these routine activities.

Sacredness. In the midst of the ordinariness, the nurses expressed a sacredness about the work. They saw their work as a privilege and a calling, as an expression of love (Lamendola, 1998, pp. 64–65).

Previously Lamendola stated that burnout occurs when the value structure of the caregiver leads to expectations that cannot be met. This view helps to explain why nurses who have let go of a concept of health that means absence of disease are able to find meaning and reward in the process of dying. The situation offers an opportunity to contemplate the meaning of living and dying and makes it possible to transcend the physical limitations of the body and experience the boundarylessness and timelessness of the human spirit.

The centrality of mutual process to the theory of HEC requires a method of study that captures the nature of the relationship. The research allows the process to unfold in a natural way.

Chapter 6

Beyond Method

. . . it is we ourselves . . . who in our own bodies are the best and most sophisticated technology there is—we are the path beyond technology.

Jose Arguelles (1987)

Bortoft (1996) reminded us that the true order of the world is found by going beyond the senses, and even sometimes by going against the established relationships. The data of my early study of time perception across the life span ran counter to the established changes in physiology regarding aging,[1] but when viewed from the standpoint of HEC, they could be seen as having new meaning (Newman, 1987). The theory does not simply rearrange parts but reveals a new meaning, which cannot be derived from the old perspective. From Bortoft: "When we recognize this transformation of the facts, we discover for ourselves the primacy of meaning . . ." (p. 160). We are seeing differently instead of seeing different things. In viewing a patient's situation, we see differently because of the difference in our concept of health.

The life sciences deal with three kinds of knowledge: the biological (sensory), the mind (symbolic), and the subtle (trans-symbolic). Knowledge of the subtle is direct and cannot be mediated by symbols (words). It grasps reality as a whole: ". . . the subtle level can never be entirely understood through the concepts, logic, and thought of the mental level. To reach such understanding requires direct access, insight, or transcendence to the subtle level" (Friedman, 1990, p. 106). But recog-

---

[1]Physiology would predict a slowing down of the biological clock with aging (diminishing perceived time per clock unit); the data indicated an expanded present (increased perceived time per clock unit).

nizing the value of each, Lindbergh (1972) viewed sensory and extrasensory information as different faces of each other. For example, refer again to Capasso's story of her patient who experienced emotional release in tears and physical relief in the loss of fluid in her leg.

Being able to see pattern is crucial to the nursing process. We usually think of numbers as quantitative, but the essence of number is qualitative, and the relationship between two numbers (a fraction) is the beginning of pattern (Muses, 1972, p. 111). On the other hand, the volume of a container (a quantitative indicator) says nothing about the quality of its contents and does not reflect pattern. Muses (p. 325) declared that "The science of quantity and the science of wholeness are incommensurable." He maintained that both are true—in that they reveal different aspects of nature—but incommensurable and, therefore, cannot be in competition with one another. The problem-solving approach in traditional nursing research is primarily quantitative, whereas the emphasis on evolving pattern is a qualitative reflection of wholeness.

A shift of axis in a geometrical figure (Fig. 6–1) is a helpful analogy to understanding situations in which clients are confronted with what seems like an immutable pattern. Sometimes all that is needed is a shift

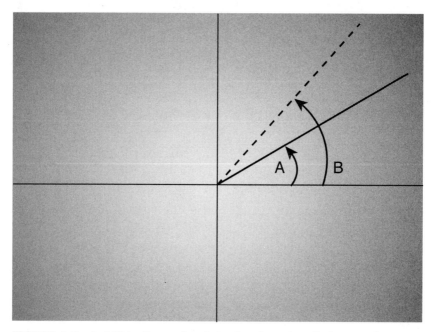

FIGURE 6–1. A shift in the angle of viewing from A to B changes the perspectives.

in the angle of viewing (like from "smoking is bad for you" to "what is important to you"). In one instance, a mother felt rejected and caged in by her adult children's choice of life style, which was contrary to her teachings. A shift in her own rigidly held values could have broadened her perspective and opened the way for mutual respect and caring.

Empiricism yields a naive accumulation of facts. Rogers (1970) rejected an inductive approach of simply gathering facts and insisted that theory came first. In the paradigm shift epitomized by Copernicus' revelation that the earth orbited the sun, by the time observational evidence confirmed his idea, the data were almost superfluous. Copernicus did not come up with new elements but a new perspective, a new organizing idea that revealed a new pattern of relationships and a new meaning. That's what happens when a nurse resonates with a patient's experience from the standpoint of health as expanding consciousness (HEC). The whole person, not the disease, is the focus of attention and the understanding is different. Here is how a young nurse described her first encounter with HEC:

> My first experience with health as expanding consciousness (HEC) began with a research project involving Hmong women with diabetes. The Hmong were U.S. allies during the Vietnam War and fled to the U.S. as refugees in 1975. I am one of these refugees myself. I can speak, read, and write Hmong. These skills had made it easy for me to do health education with the Hmong in the past: I would basically take on a prescriptive role, telling the people what they should do to regain or maintain health. My view of health was that it was something good, not to be lost, but, if one does lose it, then one must do something to get it back. Illness was always bad and was to be avoided. This mindset made it easy for me to label diabetic Hmongs who experience complications as noncompliant. This label somehow relieved me of further responsibility to these patients. However, after I had immersed myself in HEC . . . , I quickly discarded this mindset. I began to wonder if there was something in the Hmong women's lives that would teach me to be a better nurse instead of just someone who is quick to apply the label noncompliant. Thus began my journey with practicing nursing with HEC. I interviewed two Hmong women with diabetes. I asked the women, "What is the most important person or event in your life?" In the process of answering this simple question, one Hmong woman underwent a transformation, which made me feel the awesome power of HEC. This feel for the force of HEC made me undergo a transformation: I became a firm believer in its power to heal, not in the traditional sense of making illness absent, but in the sense of making life have meaning for the patient and the nurse even in the face of what we traditionally define as illness.

I shall call this woman Maisee (pseudonym). Maisee kept telling me in the first interview that she wanted to kill herself because there was nothing to live for. In the second interview, she made a 360-degree turnaround, saying she wanted to live after all. She acknowledged that she needed to care for herself and tell health-care providers what she needed. She said she wanted to live to see her children grow up. In describing this transformation, she used the word "pli" (Hmong word implying metamorphosis), likening it to a caterpillar changing into a butterfly. I asked her if she felt my presence had somehow contributed to this metamorphosis. Her reply was, "Yes." This astounding experience is what led me to truly know in my heart, soul, and mind that I had discarded my old mindset for something that is true. Although no scientific tool I know of can measure this truth, this woman and I had experienced an expansion of consciousness (Avonne Yang, personal communication).

Focus on the whole person reveals the evolving pattern. Here is a synthesis of what a number of HEC scholars had to say about participation in patterning:

Patterning is a process of recognizing and creating meaning in life. It is enduring and evolving. It is a reflection of one's relationships with the significant people in one's life and how those relationships change over time. There is a kind of order inherent in pattern that makes it recognizable but in some sense ineffable. In engaging in the evolving process with clients, we are integral to the process and cannot step outside the process. When we do take the step of describing the evolving pattern in words and diagram, the pattern may appear fixed even though we know it is a living, evolving phenomenon. The words and diagram become metaphors for the pattern—our limited way of conveying the dynamic process. The labeling of pattern with words may mask the specificity of the pattern (as happens in stereotyping). We need to attend to the exactness of the shapes and connections of the relatedness. The dialogue between the nurse and client is a meaning-making, transforming process.

[Excerpted from an online dialogue of HEC scholars]

The concept of health from the standpoint of HEC has been characterized as dialectic (Litchfield, 1999). It is continuously changing as the client's concept of health interpenetrates with the researcher-practitioner's theoretical perspective. This change is illustrated in Litchfield's relationship with a family in which disease was a major focus; both the mother and the son experienced epileptic seizures that disrupted their lives:

Their concept of health centered on a medical perspective of the causation and treatment of epilepsy, in which the father perceived that he had no part. As the nurse-client dialogue about their health circumstances unfolded, the father began to grasp the rhythmic dissonance of the patterns of a stay-at-home mother, a hyperactive son, and the fast-paced father, who was accustomed to the activity of his work world. He saw the role he could play in offering opportunities that would allow the mother the time and space to exercise her own rhythmic (transforming) pattern while providing new father-son opportunities to exercise their own patterns. A new pattern of family relating evolved, one that incorporated the medical meaning of epilepsy within a family-oriented concept of health. This insight was accomplished by the caring dialectic and pattern recognition that took place in the nurse-client dialogue . . . [which] contained statements of the nurse-researcher merged with statements from the family reflecting their emerging enlightenment (Litchfield, as reported by Newman, 2002, p. 5).

Nursing researchers no longer need to apologize for not adhering to the dictates of conventional science. Interest-free knowledge is logically impossible, and we are free to substitute explicit interest for implicit ones (Reinharz, 1983). Transformation is inherent in the theory of health as expanding consciousness (HEC). New views and insights emerge in the nurse-client dialogue. The new vision reveals a new pattern of relationships and new meaning. Insight is internal transformation, a form of action, and is a way to conceptualize the outcome of HEC praxis.

Nursing research focuses on the relational *process,* not simply the results of the process. We are active participants, not onlookers. Ordinary thinking is already too late to capture the resonance of the process. The role of the practitioner/researcher is reconceptualized from that of a privileged manipulator and translator of expert knowledge to that of a coparticipant who works with client/participants as they seek understanding of their situations. The transformative nature of dialogue is active in this process. According to Bohm (1992), thoughts cannot comprehend the implicate order; they inevitably distort reality. Only the *process* of thinking, experienced moment-to-moment, can participate in knowing the unknown. The process is *experienced*, not conceptualized. Thinking **about** reality never gets us there; our thinking **is** reality.

PARTICIPATING IN THE UNFOLDING PROCESS

De Quincey (1998) has provided an illuminating review of the psychological and philosophical literature on consciousness, from which he concludes that second-person approaches,[2] what he refers to as intersubjective, are essential to the study of consciousness. He sees this as occurring through participation and mutuality, essential factors in the nursing process. The "inter" of intersubjectivity refers to the interpenetration of participants, pointing to one person's having direct knowledge of another person's experience. (A more explicit word might be *intra*subjectivity.) How one person shows up in the other's experience means that one can learn both about the other and also oneself through this intrapersonal dialogue. Interpenetration has been illustrated as the wave interference of two phenomena, such as the interacting waves when two rocks are thrown into a lake, and the same type of phenomenon between two interacting persons, such as the nurse and the client (Newman, 1986; 1994).

In this view, consciousness involves dialogic relations between persons. The word consciousness stems from *conscientia,* meaning knowing with. DeQuincey (1998) cited the shared experience of love as an example of this "knowing with." Love is regarded as the highest level of consciousness (Bentov, 1977; Moss, 1981; Muses, 1978). It follows that intersubjectivity is a primary way of reaching this higher level.

In the process of recalling meaningful events in their lives, people tell stories that are meaning in context, patterning through time. Frank Lamendola (personal communication, 1996) related a dream he had about pattern:

> Through listening and dialogue between researcher [practitioner] and co-researcher [client], the method of pattern recognition from a unitary, transformative perspective reveals a deep knowing about a person's movement in time and space. Pattern, from this perspective, is more significant than identifying themes, in that it reflects the wholeness of a person. What's revealed through the explicate pattern seen in the narrative and pattern diagram is the implicate pattern of the whole.

The emphasis in living systems is on the quality of the relationships and the complexity of continuing change. This emphasis indicates a need to transform a static observational system (such as diagnostic categories) into ongoing patterns of relating. To do so changes the emphasis of nursing inquiry from naming to relating, and the practitioner/researcher is integral to the focus. What is studied is *the dynamics of relating.* Consciousness is not just the informational capacity of the human

---

[2]As opposed to first-person (subjective) and third-person (objective) approaches.

system at a point in time but the evolving pattern of the human-environmental system in an interconnected flux.

The process focuses on storytelling. The nursing practitioner/researcher (PR) prompts the client/participant (CP) to tell about the most meaningful moments in her or his life. This simple question may seem overwhelming to the CP at first, but when prompted to reflect on particularly meaningful events or relationships, the CP will usually think of something. It can be a current event or something in the past. Once the CP begins to tell her or his story, the CP and PR are linked in the process of telling and listening, which may be enlarged to reciprocal storytelling. Sakalys (2003) has elaborated the importance of storytelling in nursing: "In the relational narrative, each offers to the other his or her story . . . for the purpose of developing a shared narrative that becomes the foundation for joint action in the nurse-patient relationship" (p. 232). Taylor (2001) goes further: "[Stories] turn mere chronology, one thing after another, into purposeful action of plot, and thereby into meaning . . . If nothing is connected, then nothing matters . . . They help us to see how choices and events are tied together . . ." (p. 2). The narrative can restore coherence in a client's life when it has been interrupted by illness or other disruptive events. As the client's voice is heard, the unfolding pattern will be recognized. In this process of reflection and pattern recognition, the meaning emerges. Even though in HEC research reports we often describe the evolving pattern, the process is more important than the product in affirming the client's sense of self and in promoting caring relationships. From Sakalys (2003, p. 234): "Narrative understanding is caring action . . ."

A new way of seeing takes place. It is different from the analysis prevalent in medicine. Sakalys' (2003) description of the difference in these approaches bears repeating:

> When nursing practice is situated in the narrative mode, a new lens is set; how nurses relate to patients, listen, and question differ fundamentally from traditional clinical dialogue.
>
> In [medical] history taking, nurses listen with a diagnostic, pathologizing ear, listening for facts rather than for meaning. . . . the patient's story is converted into a diagnosis and a treatment plan that subsequently informs and constructs the patient's experience as an ill person. Through this social construction, the sick lose their own experience and its meaning . . . this is the voice of medicine.

Both analytic and narrative thinking are necessary for optimal care; therefore, the use of a narrative approach does not necessitate rejection of the analytic approach. It does necessitate that nursing relinquish judgmental interpretation of the facts and place the emphasis on *privileging the voice* of the client regarding the meaning of her or his situation.

TRUSTWORTHINESS OF THIS APPROACH

The onus on new paradigm researchers is to be systematic about establishing the trustworthiness of their data. For some, "the fact that pattern recognition is done as a dialogue and patterns are discerned with the participants, validity is a non-issue. People get to claim their own reality and that reality is ever changing" (Pharris, personal communication, 2006).

At any rate, there are several ways in which the validity of the research can be supported: by going back to participants with tentative results and refining them; by evidence of increased understanding and action on the part of participants; and by evidence of how the theory is altered by the data of the research (Lather, 1986). Incidentally, if it were not possible for the theory to be altered by the research, it would be a nondialectical imposition and would be inconsistent with the essence of the theory itself. Construct validity is grounded in the dialectic between the theory, the participant/client's perspective, and the researcher's involvement in practice.

These points are illustrated in much of the HEC research (Picard & Jones, 2005) by evidence of increased understanding and action of participants. Litchfield (1999), in her study of families with frequently hospitalized children, contacted participants a year later to get their permission for publication of the data and found quite unexpectedly that the incidence of hospitalization of their children (the concern of the original study) had diminished significantly. The participants in Endo et al.'s (2000) studies reported marked changes in their relationships within their families, revealing more openness and caring. Behavioral changes were apparent in other studies as well.

An unexpected finding occurred in conjunction with Rosa's (2006) implementation of a study of HEC with patients in a wound healing unit; the nurse administrator on the unit observed that the wounds of the patients in the study were healing noticeably faster than the wounds of other patients on the unit. Although healing in the traditional sense of eradication of disease is not the claim of HEC, these changes raise the question of how HEC's transformative changes are related to somatic changes. The choice to change may or may not manifest bodily changes, but the lack of bodily changes does not negate the theory because meaning may be reflected in other ways.

Ways in which the theory of HEC has been altered by the research include: placing the emphasis on the process of patterning (Litchfield, 1999); and initiating the nurse-client encounter at the height of the client's period of uncertainty (Endo, 1998; Noveletsky-Rosenthal, 1996; Pharris, 2002), consistent with the supporting theory (Mishel, 1990; Prigogine, 1976). Although caring was not explicitly incorporated in the theory of HEC initially, as transformation in the clients' lives occurred, caring became evident in the nature of the nurse-client relationships and in the clients' subsequent relationships within their own configurations (Butrin, 1992; Endo, 1998; Litchfield, 1999; Kiser-Larson, 2002; Neill, 2002b; Pharris, 2002). These results brought about an elaboration of the relationship between knowing and caring as integral to the theory (Newman, 2002a). The continuous change inherent in the dialectical process strengthens the theory's relevance to practice.

Of note, other elaborations of the theory have been suggested by recent research. Neill (2002a) has made a distinction between the concepts of turning point and choice point, stating that there could be a number of turning points related to events in a person's life, but that this does not constitute a choice point until persons actually make a choice to change their life. I would suggest that at each turning point, a choice is immanent. Some choices may be more silent than others, such as the choice **not** to act.

EXPERIENCING PATTERN

Being known is a higher stage of development for an individual and facilitates coming into presence. Thus in the process of knowing the client, the nurse is the means by which clients actualize as a higher stage of themselves. From the experience of a nurse-researcher:

> "[The HEC] method was my primary method and I have to say it was magnificent. Indeed the HEC focus is research as praxis and that was very important to me. I interviewed cancer patients (a number of whom were close to death) and it was important to me that their participation offer them something of significance. Indeed, it did—it was transforming for me as well as the participants—and I feel that my practice will be forever changed from this experience. . . . We

modified or validated the pattern together and reflected on the meaning of pattern and the meaning of the experience we shared. The engagement with participants was powerful and important. HEC offered a valuable and highly relevant focus—the discussions generally were animated and energizing for the participants and me—the level of energy at times was surprising because many of the participants were very sick. They described to me the value for them of reflecting on their lives and their patterns. The method is indeed beautiful and powerful" (Barron, 2001).

Bortoft (1996, p. 161) repeated Goethe's maxim that "the greatest art in theoretical and practical life consists in changing a problem into a postulate." Insight derived in this way is not an inference from phenomena (an inductive approach), but a step of creative *imagination;* that is, not what causes this phenomenon but rather what meaning it has in terms of the whole. This way of seeing transcends the situations in which persons find themselves. Failure to see beyond is only a matter of limiting one's imagination (Neill, 2002b).

Research often yields data that do not confirm or falsify the theory of HEC. In such cases, we need to look beyond a particular focus to the bigger picture. For instance, one may not be able to identify evidence of expanding consciousness when looking only at the "identified" patient. A broadened view, however, of the family and community, may reveal this phenomenon. The story of Aaron's legacy (Newman, 1994), as told by the parents to Nurse Practitioner Tommet, illustrated the pivotal position of a developmentally disabled child in the transforming relationships within his family and community. Aaron was severely disabled and had frequent seizures following fetal distress at birth. His parents experienced the shock and sorrow of realizing there was something wrong with their newborn child. The first 6 months they were in a constant struggle seeking medical help and dealing with the uncertainty of his condition. In addition, they had the difficult job of finding someone to care for Aaron to give them some respite from the constant struggle. After the first year, with support systems in place, the parents began to reach out to others in the community. They decided to have two additional children, whose relationship with Aaron convinced the mother to lead in the establishment of school programs that were integrated with children with and without disabilities. She regarded this program as part of Aaron's legacy:

I think that Aaron taught our family a lot about this issue of belonging and being part of a community. Aaron's short life . . . in some ways he was much more powerful than me in being able to facilitate some changes just in attitudes by his presence. And that despite the tragedy and sorrow of his situation, I value what he gave to us . . . (Newman, 1994, p. 27).

Aaron's story illustrates the pattern of the whole as it expanded from individual to family to community. There were no separate parts.

The purpose of nursing research is to inform nursing practice as fully as possible. Attention to the pattern and quality of relationships becomes the experience of nursing practice in terms of itself. The researcher learns to surrender to the process: "When the will becomes receptive, then consciousness becomes participative" (Bortoft, 1996, p. 242). In contrast, when the will is assertive the researcher/practitioner is separated from the phenomenon as onlooker. Lamendola was specific about the need to relinquish his assertiveness by giving up his agenda while interacting with men who were HIV positive (Lamendola & Newman, 1994):

> I needed to let go of thinking I had to lead the interview in a direction or make the pain better or fix a problem. The purpose . . . was to allow a sense of the whole to emerge (p. 20).

Goethe sought to make the pattern of the phenomenon visible, not to explain it:

> Far from being onlookers, detached from the phenomenon, or at most manipulating it externally, Goethean scientists are engaged with it in a way which entails their own development. . . . [S]ensorial imagination is not sitting there waiting to be activated. It has to be *developed*, and this is done by practicing . . . (Bortoft, 1996, p. 245).

The involvement of practicing nurses in pattern recognition with patients with cancer (Endo, Miyahara, Suzuki, and Ohmasa, 2005) and of nursing students in pattern recognition of their own patterns (Endo, personal communication) are examples of the development of this skill. We must seek transformative learning experiences that will prepare students for this essential task of resonating and using their imaginal knowledge. For nursing scientists, questions often arise regarding which instruments are unitary in nature. The answer is that the scientist herself or himself is the instrument. This seeing **is** the theory: the experience of insight.

When we shift from being an onlooker to being a participant in the health experience of the client, we reach a different understanding. The "conversation" is a synergistic condition in which each becomes more fully oneself through the other. This occurs when nurses work with clients within the context of health as expanding consciousness. Both the nurse and the client become more fully themselves and experience a higher stage of their own being. This is the path beyond technology.

A willingness to be transformed is an essential characteristic of the participating scientist.

Willis Harman, 1988

Chapter 7

Transforming Nursing Education

A true meeting of the minds is a transformative event.
Christian de Quincey, 2005

The discipline of nursing provides the foundation for nursing education. The increasing emphasis on the unitary, transformative paradigm, as introduced by Rogers (1970), focuses on the process of the nurse-client relationship. It has led to the development of a number of theories that emanate from a unified philosophical perspective. The task for educators is to ground nursing education in the discipline while at the same time offering relevant knowledge from other disciplines. David Peat (1991), physicist and philosopher, has offered a philosophy of wholeness that is consistent with the unitary, transformative perspective in nursing and warned, "If we are to move toward a more holistic and healthy world, then we must discover a way of unifying the statements of objective science with our personal vision of the world, and we must do this without diluting the authenticity of either approach" (p. 47). Whereas health knowledge from other disciplines has dominated our curricula in the past, we now face the task of integrating that knowledge within the context of the unitary, transformative framework of nursing. Attention to the nature of transformative learning will help to establish the priorities of the discipline.

TRANSFORMATIVE LEARNING

Inherent in transformative learning is the expansion of consciousness: Transformative learning has been defined as "the expansion of consciousness in any human system through the transformation of basic worldview and specific capacities of the self . . ." [It involves] "a transformed capacity for thinking, transformed to be more dialectical . . . thinking (for example) that perceives polarities as mutually creative resources rather than as exclusive and competitive options" (Elias, 1997, p. 3, 3–4). This way of thinking is important in seeing variations in theory as complementary with one another rather than competitive. It includes ways of thinking that include both the intellectual and intuitive. It is a participative approach to thinking and learning.

The conditions for transformative learning are first and foremost *relational:* an interpersonal context that provides affective support and ensures that all participants have equal access to information and processes of information exchange. There must be personal capacities of awareness and discernment, and the flexibility to approach some learning appreciatively, some critically, and the wisdom to know the difference (Elias, 1997). Transformative learning is important in shifting from an observer mode to a participant mode of inquiry. In an observer mode, one can easily interpret evidence in a way that fits one's existing frame of reference; in transformative learning, the structure of consciousness itself is changed from a perspective that is static to a process-based consciousness that is dynamic and evolving (Tang, 1997). It is experiential; the learner is sensitive to both her or his own feelings and also to the feelings of others.

Study is part of an intense process of personal transformation. Along with a shift in the collective consciousness of the nursing profession, we need integration of personal transformation in the nursing curriculum. This involves both subject matter and subtle resonance arising in the learning circles. The study of the universe "out there" is also seeing patterns "in here." The stronger and clearer the focus, the more likely that skillful inquiry will spark deep changes in people's lives. Chris Bache (undated, p. 5), director of transformational learning at the Institute of Noetic Science, sees transformational learning as a playful dance of content and resonance: To be aligned with one's truth "is to be aligned with reality, and alignment opens oneself to the healing, insight, and transformation that is continuously flowing from the whole to its many parts." Only the *process* of thinking, experienced moment-to-moment, is open to knowing the unknown.

In transpersonal learning, the teacher and students are not separate objects in the transfer of knowledge. As the teacher's consciousness is expanded, students will experience it by way of resonance. Teaching becomes a direct engagement of intuitive awareness. Bache (2000) pointed to an example of resonance in the classroom when the teacher pauses in search of the right example to communicate a difficult concept, a pause that constitutes an opportunity for intuition to transform the situation into a creative direction instead of a predictable loop. Students in Bache's classes reported experiencing intimate connections to their lives and he asked, "What were these powerful processes that were linking me to them in such an intimate fashion without either of us soliciting the connection?" (p. 190). He explained this in terms of the resonance occurring in the oneness of all, adding that "Separate minds are an illusion of the senses" (p. 195).

Bache recognized the synchronicity of teacher-student experiences and student-student experiences as "symptoms of a unified learning field" (p. 195). He cited Sheldrake's concept of morphic fields, which predicts that once a field is formed from, say, a new thought, it is easier for that new learning to take place in subsequent times. So courses that are taught on a repeated basis have distinct morphic fields, or learning fields, in which discoveries are cumulative. My experience of teaching a new course was that I had to teach it several times before it came together as a meaningful whole. Each year that a course is taught, the field (a combination of the course mind and the class mind) becomes stronger. This cumulative effect is apparent in the readiness and ease of understanding with which current students embrace nursing theory compared with the difficulties of earlier students.

One of the goals for transformative learning, as suggested by Watson-Gegeo (2005), is seeing the teacher as a catalyst to help students become who they will become rather than be "trained." Grand (2005) added the need to enable students to develop capacities for feeling, expression, and self-reflection. Nursing educators are incorporating a variety of ways to do this as they teach the theory of HEC. In order to learn pattern recognition in a relational context, one must experience the transformation that accompanies the shift in paradigm. One assignment that has been effective in bringing students to this realization is composed of having students select a willing participant for this interactive process and follow the directions included in the praxis protocol (See Appendix A). The revelation of the unfolding pattern is transforming. They begin to see the whole person, not just manifestations of a disease.

Jones, an experienced teacher of HEC, has shared an assignment that she has found meaningful in helping students experience the shift in paradigm:

> I have students first use a problem-solving approach to understand the person. They assess an experience using a functional health pattern framework and generate the content of the experience with some conclusions; that is, medical or nursing diagnoses. Then they shift the paradigm and use the HEC process dialogue in an encounter with the same patient and follow the praxis approach to identify pattern, and . . . Wow! . . . The experience is transformative. What emerges is new insight for the person: Discovery of the importance of pattern, witnessing change through self recognition, choice/change, and personal awareness of the student's role in partnership. Later in the semester, when students dialogue about a patient, it is not uncommon to hear students comment, "What you need to do with this patient situation is 'shift' the paradigm" (Jones, personal communication).

A third way of promoting transformative learning has been demonstrated by Endo et al. (2007) in their involvement of students in a project of pattern recognition with the students themselves as the participants and faculty as the facilitators of the process. The HEC praxis approach was used, and students and faculty jointly considered the tapes of the conversations and what they meant in terms of the students' patterns. Again, the process was transformative in the students' relationships with each other and with their families. Other lifestyle changes occurred.

All of the previous ways of experiencing the deep interpersonal relationship with another help students realize the paradigm shift from outer knowledge to inner knowledge of the whole. The essential nature of this type of learning to practice makes it imperative that it be started early in the nursing curriculum, so that the link between theory and practice permeates throughout the clinical experiences. Repeatedly I receive e-mails from students who have just discovered the relevance of nursing theory, as a senior or a graduate student, and they ask, "**Why wasn't this taught from the beginning?**"

What is the nature of education that will prepare a professional with knowledge and abilities to deal with the uncertainties of multiple health situations? Montuori's (2006) recommendation for a program of transformative learning would integrate more traditional education (which he saw as reproductive of the existing social and academic order) with an intuitive approach to accomplish what he calls creative inquiry. His classifications stem from a dichotomy of an old paradigm/new paradigm view of part versus whole, quantitative versus qualitative, logic versus intuition, and so on. A creative inquiry approach would emphasize connection (rather than separation) and dialectical thinking. To get to this point would require the incorporation of the complexity of paradox and asymmetry. It would cultivate tolerance for ambiguity to do well in situations where there is no set way of doing things—no clear guidelines in a field where there are multiple and at times conflicting perspectives. Creative inquirers can develop new ways of making meaning and explore situations without premature closure. They are more comfortable with uncertainties and are trusting of the knowledge from within. These characteristics are important for nurses who "hang in there" with clients in the uncertainty of their transforming trajectories. They are "in the moment" and responsive to the uniqueness of the person and situation.

Part of pattern recognition is being able to look at things from a different point of view, a reframing of the situation by shifting the angle of viewing. The ability to do this is facilitated by a preference for asymmetry, which may lead to new insights. From Montuori (2006, p. 12), "Complexity, asymmetry, disorder, the unknown, the unexplained, and the edges of the paradigm become a source of stimulation and possibility . . ." For students, the challenge is to develop their tolerance for uncertainty as they develop their own voice. In contrast, attempts to maintain equilibrium are associated with closed views and stereotypes, which block the insight one is seeking.

Montuori's experience in establishing a new frame of reference included asking students to reflect on their own educational experience. They were asked what they aspired to be, immersed in the historical development of the field, and stimulated to envision the possibilities that lie ahead in the field. He suggested that jazz is a good metaphor for this type of education, combining the creative collaboration of highly skilled players who both support and challenge their colleagues: "This involves the ability to integrate the various aspects of one's being to be present in the moment with as much of oneself as one can bring to bear on the moment" (p. 18). It means bringing all of oneself to the inquiry, biases and all. One nurse has pointed out in the framework of being open to the experience, she is able to utilize herself totally in the process: "I bring everything I can (who I am, my experiences, the fact that I'm a mother) to the process—it's not only okay, it's important!" (Newman, Lamb, & Michaels, 1991, p. 406). This type of learning integrates rigor and imagination, discipline and improvisation, grounding in knowledge and creative speculation. Not-knowing becomes an ally.

This type of education is foundational to nursing practice within the context of HEC. Both nurses who practice relatively independently and those who practice primarily in the realm of delegated medical tasks have a responsibility to focus their relationship with the patient on the meaning of their evolving pattern. The medical concerns may be the nurse's point of access to the client; the meaning of the presenting pattern is the opening for transformation.

According to Bache (2000), the key ingredients for these fields to form are (1) collective intention focused on group projects, (2) a project of sustained duration, and (3) repetition of the project in the same form many times. The higher the quality of engagement between students and course material, the greater and more lasting the learning. Nursing courses lend themselves readily to these criteria. For example, Gail Lindsay's graduate nursing course, Patterns in the Health Experience of Older Persons, which focuses on the theory of health as expanding consciousness, is exemplary of the essentials of transformative learning (Personal communication). It integrates the intellectual and the intuitive by containing sufficient theoretical content from the literature to relate to others from more traditional learning environments and requires in-depth experiences regarding the meaning these approaches have in the students' own lives and their relationships to others. Picard and Mariolis (2005) too provided opportunities for students through group and student-teacher interaction to express the meaning in their own lives. Bronson (2006, p. 2), when introducing the topic of transformative learning, asserted that ". . . action is always informed by theory, and theory is viewed as a form of practice." The demands of nursing practice are such that integration of theory and practice is a priority in nursing education.

Transformative learning can be experienced in a group. The Bohmian dialogue is a way to experience group consciousness, a way for a group to think and feel together, to explore the spontaneous unfolding of meaning, to pay attention to the feelings of our bodies (Bohm, 1992). The HEC scholars group has engaged in dialogue on a number of occasions for this purpose, to think beyond the boundaries of one's own perspective, to move on to further horizons. The dialogue begins in silence and proceeds without a leader. Whatever surfaces, is the substance of dialogue. Only one person speaks at any time. Nothing is off limits; yet we do not speak to force a point. We listen openly, suspending evaluation and judgment. The purpose of dialogue is not to provide answers or solutions or actions. It is simply to explore consciousness. We are invited to listen for the meaning of every communication. It is about being in relationship (Bohm, 1992; DeQuincey, 2005). A kind of group mind is always trying to happen in order to make coherent what is incoherent: "It is the awakening of humanity as a whole that is the current project of history; nothing less will satisfy the Creative Principle" (Bache, 2000, p. 181).

DEVELOPMENT OF THE DISCIPLINE

Selection of which theories are integrated in practice and the timing of when they are introduced in the curriculum becomes an issue. Answers to these questions lie in our understanding of the nature of the discipline, how it is developing, and how our practice is actualized. In my concern about connecting to others committed to a unitary, transformative paradigm of health and nursing, I have found Peat's (1991) thoughts on the order of the world relevant to the development of the discipline of nursing and have juxtaposed my thoughts as follows:

From Peat	**Relevance to Nursing**
A collective is held together by bonds of attraction between units, not by any one person or persons.	The discipline of nursing is held together by the connections between theories, not by the theorists themselves.
Each unit is free to act locally, but there is a collective dance that all participate in nonlocally.	There is an overall pattern of the discipline revealed in the many specific applications of theory at the local level.
This takes on a specific global form that each subsystem fits into and guides the continuing growth of the organism.	These theoretical patterns fit into a larger pattern that defines the discipline and guides our developing practice.

continued

continued

From Peat	Relevance to Nursing
There is an early ambiguous state composed of a combination of different states, superimposed on each other. Then at some critical point, the superimposed wave function collapses into a definite form, and from then on, the organism will develop according to a particular global pattern.	Nursing has been through an ambiguous state of multiple, competing, possibly disconnected theories. The discipline is at a critical point of an emerging, overarching form that will direct its continuing development.
At this point, the thing that holds the organism together is not the initial strong bonds of attraction between units, but the additional, smaller attractions (like the weak energy field) that orchestrates the whole.	The nature of the overall pattern of nursing knowledge goes beyond the initial links to emerge as a unified whole.
It is not the strength of the interaction that matters but its very special form.	It is not the specific connections that make the difference but the pattern of the whole.

We have begun to put it all together as a structure of the discipline (Roy & Jones, 2007). From my perspective, key connecting points include: mutual process, caring presence, pattern recognition, resonance with the information of the whole, and expanding consciousness. As the pattern of the whole continues to generate new order, other connecting points will emerge.

COMING HOME

I am encouraged that nurses who had become disillusioned by a lack of a truly nursing perspective in their practice have come "home" to nursing and are reexperiencing the joy of nursing practice. Recently a nurse who has become acquainted with the theory of HEC posted on the

Web site[1] dialogue: "I have not felt this alive about my work in nursing ever . . . and I have always loved nursing." Falkenstern (2003) eloquently expressed what the shift to HEC meant to her as she reentered a world of nursing practice and education after a 10-year hiatus:

> As I rediscovered the nursing world after my return to nursing practice and education after an absence of ten years to raise my children, I felt discouraged when I learned of the current status of nurses and nursing. . . . However, my experience with this study [with families who have a child with special health-care needs] has rekindled my passion for nursing. I felt affirmed that . . . a movement is growing to recapture the essence and value of nursing. . . . I realized that a nurse can experience joy and renewed energy by choosing to practice nursing within health as expanding consciousness.
>
> From my personal experience with the families in this study, I realized that by practicing according to this theory, the nurse does not just treat a person's illness or disease but pays attention to the whole person and helps them to see the pattern and meaning of their experience in their current, often challenging situation. . . .
>
> . . . I realized that a nurse can practice health as expanding consciousness whether the interaction between the nurse and the patient is very brief or long term. The nurse can communicate that s/he is *being "wholly" with* the client while *doing* regular tasks *for* that client, such as taking vital signs, checking IVs, and giving medications. That is, the nurse can fully interact with the person as a human being. While burnout has often been cited as a reason not to get "too involved" with patients, I found that the practice of nursing within health as expanding consciousness, on a more personal level, can be energizing. During my nurse-family interaction in this study, I saw persons gain insight into their lives, let go of guilt, and find new ways to structure their interactions with others.
>
> My experience with the families in this study was a personal journey that touched my heart—and gave me hope . . . Their strength in the face of challenges, discouragement, and prejudice amazed me. When I asked one family how they kept their hope and carried on, their reply summarized an energy that was present in all the families, "It's love. With love anything is possible." As nurses, we carry a special charge, to attend to our patients, as human to human, with love (Falkenstern, 2003, pp. 232–233).

---

[1]www.healthasexpandingconsciousness.org

Chapter 8

A Transforming Arc

. . . nursing is in a position to shape the future stage of evolution of the universe.

Sister Callista Roy, 2007

For us to participate fully and creatively in shaping our future, we need to better understand the underlying patterns and influences of our collective past.

Richard Tarnas, 2002

A s our global civilization becomes increasingly dysfunctional and we face the possibility of catastrophe, we need to examine the contrasting myths prevalent in Western thinking regarding the evolution of consciousness. The most familiar one is that of an extraordinary journey from ignorance and suffering to a world of increasing knowledge and well-being—an onward and upward direction seen as progressive emancipation. The other view is that of humanity's fall and separation from oneness with nature, as seen in exploitation of nature, devastation of indigenous cultures, and spiritual emptiness. What we need to recognize is that both underlie and inform each other. The subject-object divide upon which science was founded seeks to rule out human projections such as meaning and purpose. In contrast, meaning and purpose are seen in the primal worldview as permeating the world with the same resonant reality, flowing between inner and outer without absolute distinction. When there is a confrontation between the two, the intellect wins. The drive for money and power and technological superiority supersedes other aspirations. But fortunately the post-Copernican and post-Cartesian shifts in paradigm hold that the primary datum of human experience is human experience itself and is reflective of the underlying forms and patterns of the world. We have the potential for a new participatory wholeness (Tarnas, 2002).

Developmental principles, such as those suggested by Ken Wilber's (1998) integral theory, take us beyond our usual view that expanding consciousness is always upward and outward. A more inclusive perspective embraces an involutional development that emphasizes a nondual ground of being in which transcendence is balanced by a descending force that integrates and heals. The movement toward progress and domination is balanced by moving inward and experiencing wholeness. Wilber's position is that human development covers a large range of evolutionary territory, both individual and collective, and involves a process of evolution to higher transcendent structures that is complementary with involution to more fundamental levels of compassion and spirit (Edwards, 2002). Bache (2000), from the perspective of his personal experience in holotropic therapy, supports this larger trajectory of evolution/involution. He described the involutionary phase as the "dark night of the soul," an experience in which we must "let fall from us everything that we thought we were or thought we needed" before reaching a new understanding of the interconnectedness of all life (pp. 15–16). Kidd's (1996) journey from a life engulfed in patriarchy to one in touch with the feminine spirit within involved a descent into the darkness of her soul before emerging as an integrated self.

When I first started working on this book, I was rejoicing in the opening of East and West with the crumbling of the Berlin wall. I was reveling in the prospect of no boundaries between countries and ideologies. Then in the last 5 years I have been stymied by the seemingly insurmountable barriers between nations/people/ideologies, even within my own country. In the aftermath of the 9/11/01 attack on the World Trade Center and the Pentagon, I, along with people all over the world, searched for a way to respond. As a people, we were shocked . . . angry . . . afraid. Now we have experienced even greater loss of life and disruption as a result of the natural disasters on the U.S. Gulf Coast, in Indonesia, Pakistan, the continuing violence in the Mideast, the poverty and violence of African nations, and the seeming inabilities of our governments to cope with them. The predictions in the 1980s of massive physical disruptions are unfolding before our eyes: *We Are the Earthquake Generation* (Goodman, 1979; Newman, 1995b). We are left with trying to find meaning and understanding to guide the transformation of our society. Deeply embedded in the hearts of many of our fellow world citizens are frustration and hatred; for some, deprivation and helplessness; for others who have been protected from the ravages of poverty and war, indifference. Capitalism appeared to triumph over Communism in the late 20th century, but now in the early years of the 21st century, some are seeking to find a way to share the world's wealth. The blow to the economy compels it. The awakening of our conscience demands it.

There is a need for a spiritual rebirth of our world, but as Bache (2000) asserted, we must experience a death of the old ways first. Bache cited Grosso's claim that the specter of global death may be fueling profound psychic transformation. Other major thinkers in terms of the global crisis regard the evolution of the human species as nearing a breakthrough (Elgin, 2002–2003; Russell, 1992). Bache (2000, p. 224) described the "dawn" of his own experience as becoming comfortable with the loss of boundaries—of race, socioeconomic distinctions, nationality, religion—with the question, "What would it take for the whole of humanity to make this quantum jump in awareness?" What dies during the dark night of the soul is our deep attachment to separateness itself.

Friedman (2005) has chronicled the convergence of computerization, subsequent worldwide collaboration of new business practices, and the opening up of information and opportunity to millions the world over in what he refers to as the flattening of the world, a horizontal playing field. It is mind-boggling to consider this transformation. Is it a manifestation of the harmonic convergence predicted by Arguelles (1987) two decades ago?

Is the thesis of expanding consciousness on shaky ground? In assuming that life (and health) are moving inextricably toward expanded consciousness, it is important to remember that the theory of HEC encompasses disruptions and what might be considered downturns as manifestations of expanding consciousness. Confidence in open boundaries in the face of disaster was not misplaced; it just requires a greater *imagination* as to how it will unfold. The process of expanding consciousness is the process of awakening the divine in participants (Fox, 1988).

The disciplines of medicine and nursing have represented different cultures—one of curing and one of caring. They have evolved in different directions. Much of the talent and ingenuity of nursing has been focused on disease care rather than people care. Yet lying beneath the instrumental focus is the traditional mission of nursing to be present with persons in the transitional experiences of their lives. That purpose is yearning to express itself in ways that allow the wholeness of clients to emerge in unimagined ways, as evidenced in the Picard and Jones (2005) creative work, *Giving Voice to What We Know.* There is a need for a transforming vision of our disciplines' collective commitments. For a cultural death to occur, there must be a loss of deeply held ways of viewing each other and the collapse of deeply embedded intellectual paradigms (Bache, 2000). There must be a shift in the way we feel about each other. The larger truth of our relationships is that of interpenetration as partners in the complex dance of health care.

Bache (2000) points out that the Western project of the last 4000 years has been largely a masculine enterprise of autonomy, rationality, and separation from nature. The cost has been repression of the feminine dimension. He cites Tarnas as recognizing the emergence of the feminine, not only in the growing empowerment of women, but also in a multitude of characteristics such as increasing unity with nature, increasing embrace of human community, valuing partnership, and the urge to reconnect the body and emotions, imagination and intuition. Interesting also is the rising appreciation of hermeneutics and other nonobjectivist epistemologies and of scientific theories of the holonomic universe. These changes indicate a spiritual rebirth of humanity taking place. It is an opportunity for us as nurses to stand in the center of our truth and be fully present in the evolving health-care arena.

There is evidence of the coming together of mind and heart in the work of varied health scientists. We are entering into something new, and we cannot know where it is headed, but we can know that the way to get there is by expanding our ways of knowing to include a dialectical synthesis of world and self. Tarnas (2002, p. 10) urged:

> . . . our task is to develop a moral and aesthetic imagination deep enough and wide enough to encompass the contradictions of the time and of our history, the tremendous loss and tragedy as well as greatness and nobility; an imagination capable of recognizing that where there is light there is shadow, that out of hubris and fall can come moral regeneration, out of suffering and death, resurrection and rebirth.

As we picture our planet Earth spiraling through our solar system, we can see that there is no up or down. One way does not exist without the other—the pathway of each arc is completed by the other. Nursing's history of complementing medicine, long seen as subordinate, can now be viewed as a transforming, healing, integrating presence.

This is my message to nurses and others in the health-care arena: **imagine** a world of caring, sharing, and creativity in conjunction with continuing scientific breakthroughs. Summon the courage to act on that imagination. Remember the power of an idea! Just as the flutter of butterfly wings can be felt around the world, so the actions of one person can start a transforming avalanche in health care. In Friedman's words, the small can act big and have tremendous influence (Friedman, 2005).

What the world needs now is connectedness. There is a need for a global network that is multicultural, multidimensional. It is centered in individual and local partnerships and is always shifting, changing, open to new perspectives. Nursing is in a position to facilitate such a network. Our tradition of caring, nurturance, and understanding of love as the highest level of consciousness makes it possible for nursing to be the connecting link in the needed reformulization of the health-care system as one of cooperation, collaboration, and partnership.

The underlying implicate order of nursing's mission—caring in the human health experience—is the transforming pattern. In the unfolding of it, we are its transforming presence.

HECPraxis: The Process of Pattern Recognition

Praxis involves the merging of *a priori* theory, research, and practice. Health as expanding consciousness (HEC) provides the theoretical orientation. The nurse must come to the encounter with an understanding of the theory of HEC, which is embodied and pervasive from the very beginning. The following steps were developed primarily for research purposes, but the elements of the process are the same for practice. More specificity is usually required in recording data for research; the meetings are usually audiotaped, and precautions regarding research with human subjects must be taken.

Engaging with the client/participant (CP)   The intent is for the nurse to be fully present with the client in terms of what is most meaningful to the client. At the initial meeting the practitioner/researcher (PR) asks the client/participant (CP) to describe the most meaningful events and persons in her or his life. This question may be modified to fit the particular circumstances. If the CP needs help in thinking of something considered important, the PR may prompt the CP to think of something from childhood that stands out in memory. This is a story-telling activity that is guided by the CP and proceeds in a nondirective manner. The PR participates by being an active listener and clarifies and reflects as relevant. The emphasis is on the unfolding pattern of the CP's life, but the PR is free to reciprocate by telling her or his own story as deemed appropriate. Occasionally more direct questions are offered. In being fully present in the moment, the PR will be sensitive to intuitive hunches about what to say or ask.

Sometimes, based on experience of traditional interviewing, the PR thinks it is necessary to "collect data," that is, get information. Rather, the need is to *interact authentically* with the CP. In other instances, the PR may ask what is meaningful to the CP but be unable to accept what the CP is saying because it is not somehow what the PR is looking for. So there is no follow-up, and often another question is asked, most often for factual type information. *It is not necessary to gather information.* The objective of this interaction is to grasp **meaning.** It is important to stay with whatever the person says no matter how insignificant it may seem at the time. Fortunately the CP will keep the dialogue on target if the PR will allow it. There is no sense of direction other than that offered by the CP. The end point of the encounter comes as a natural pause, a feeling that there is some closure to the line of thinking.

Development of the narrative   The PR notes the statements deemed most important to the CP and arranges them in chronological order to form a narrative trajectory of the most significant relationships. Natural breaks where a pattern shift occurs are noted and form the basis of sequential configurations of relationships, which begin to reveal the evolving pattern.

It has been found helpful to transmute the narrative to a simple diagram illustrating the sequential configurations of relationships and meaningful events. The nature of the pattern of person-environment interactions are characterized in terms of the flow of relatedness; for example, blocked, diffuse, disorganized, repetitive, loving, abusive, giving, receiving, or whatever descriptors and metaphors come to mind. As the pattern begins to emerge, CPs have commented that the diagrammatic portrayal helps them to see the evolving pattern all at once. Some PRs prefer to share a written narrative with the clients for them to read at their leisure.

Follow-up meeting(s)   The PR and CP meet again, and the PR shares the data with the CP without interpretation. It simply is a portrayal of the CP's story and accentuates the contrasts and repetitions in relationships over time. This mutual viewing is an opportunity for the CP to affirm and clarify or revise the story being portrayed. If the PR is in doubt about any aspect of the story, now is the time to clarify. As the PR and CP reflect together on the CP's life pattern, the CP may express signs that pattern recognition is occurring (or has already occurred in the interval following the first meeting). Either of the participants may want to proceed with additional reflections in subsequent meetings until no further insight is reached.

Most researchers consider that a minimum of three meetings is needed. Sometimes no signs of pattern recognition emerge, and that, too, is meaningful in terms of the lack of an observable pattern for the person. It is not to be forced.

Application of the theory   Inherent in the nature of praxis is the fact that the theory is active throughout the encounter. Postencounter analysis will include more intense examination in relation to the theory of health as expanding consciousness and may include comparison to supporting theorists' work (e.g., Bohm, Prigogine, Young) and other nursing theories, such as uncertainty (Mishel) and transcendence (Reed, 1991). Transformational changes that occur for both the CP and the PR are noted.

Family and community pattern   Once patterns of individuals are identified, the reciprocal pattern of their environment, their relationships to family and community, become apparent. For example, when students drop out of school, what role do family and school officials play in this loss? When a woman feels isolated and caged within her own home, what is the reciprocal pattern among her family? Pharris (2005) has used this means of identifying community health patterns with verification in the form of dialogue among community participants. In her study of adolescents who had committed murder, she found "not a common pattern of pathologically disturbed youth, but rather a common pattern of interaction" with their community (Pharris, 2002).

Appendix B

Questions and Commentary[1]

Was there one defining moment or event that led you to formulate your theory?

I don't think there was any one defining moment regarding the formulation of the theory, but many along the way: My experience with my mother's illness before entering nursing; my study with Martha Rogers; my fascination with the concepts of movement, time, space and consciousness as I worked with rehab patients; and importantly, the opportunity to present the theory at a 1978 conference, which compelled me to put it all together. And, of course, it is still developing via the many scholars who have responded to the challenge.

Were there any other theorists besides Rogers who had a large influence on your work?

Dorothy Johnson's early work (1961) on "The Significance of Nursing Care" was an inspiration to me when I was a senior nursing student. It declared that the knowledge of nursing was different from the knowledge of medicine—something I had sensed in my beginning practice. I continued to correspond with her after I engaged on my path of theory development in nursing. Also, Itzhak Bentov's conceptualization of consciousness (1977) helped me to articulate what I was beginning to understand about the consciousness of the whole.

If the medical community followed your theory, do you think we could avoid many of the illnesses of our time?

That may be a possibility, but that's not the intent of the theory, which is to embrace the unfolding pattern of the whole whatever it is and grow with it.

---

[1]Excerpted from the Dialogue page of www.healthasexpandingconsciousness.org Comments are provided by M. Newman unless otherwise indicated.

How do you feel about the idea of your theory as a spiritual component or explanation of religious orientation?

I don't think of the theory as spiritual or an explanation of religious orientation, but I agree with you that it strongly resonates with multiple religious beliefs throughout the world. Perhaps that's what higher consciousness is.

What do you see as the role of nursing?

The nurse enters into a caring relationship of pattern recognition that makes it possible for clients to understand the meaning of their experience and find their own way in the health process of expanding consciousness.

What does the discipline need most from the current new generation of nurses?

A commitment to the knowledge of the discipline and engaging in practice guided by nursing theory.

What is your advice to novices?

Trust in the knowledge that comes from within, and be open to new perspectives, such as seeing the pattern of the community as a reciprocal of the individual pattern.

What would you say to encourage the students just starting out in a nursing program?

"Stand in the center of your truth" (from Jose Arguelles). What this statement means to me is that each of us has access to the truth of the universe, and if we open ourselves to it, it will guide us in our relationships with each other and with our patients.

In the current fast-paced practice settings where the time spent with patients is often short and is spent performing tasks that are more medically based, what can be said or done in just a few minutes?

It is not a matter of what you say or do, but what you feel. If you are open to what is most meaningful to the patient, it will be felt. This type of communication (which I sometimes refer to as resonance) is like a wave phenomenon. It occurs instantly and does not require verbal communication. It is being open to information that you receive rather intuitively.

From a respondent (3/14/06): One of the simplest examples of using your theory in practice is recognizing that persons are more complex than the symptoms they present with, and that their illness is just one manifestation of their life and their interaction with their environment (rhythmic fluctuation, order/disorder). While multitasking, I try to create space to reflect on what is meaningful to them. I frequently ask patients what they do/did for a living, what they are passionate about, what worries them most about their experience, shifting the focus on **exploration rather than on repair**, and indirectly make them aware that we aren't trying to make them whole, because **they already are whole**, and experts in their own care. I don't try to prescribe a set of actions, but offer options that they can decide on. One lady, as she was telling her story, stopped to thank me for listening, "most people don't ask." **I work in an ER/ICU setting, and even with these brief or limited encounters, it's amazing the patterns that emerge,** (family dynamics, self image, moments of disruption beyond or contributing to the present illness) and how enlightening it is to see the connections that can be made. In making sense of their circumstances, and trying to find new answers that work for the given situation, their needs may become clear, and nurses are in a position to offer resources from the wider community. **By caring, which doesn't take much time but does require intentionality, the transformational experience is also mine.** Even when the connections or patterns aren't clear, I try to be open to the potential for transformation in every encounter. Through HEC I'm more aware of and subtly try to remind my patients of our situational freedom: we may not be able to change the situation, but we can change our attitude about it, the uncertainty of it.

Do you feel these (short-span relationships) are the times when the family of the patients could be the focus of pattern recognition and expanding consciousness?

The family (or lack thereof) is always considered in the overall pattern of the patient and may present a crucial opening for insight and action to occur. It is not necessarily the focus in situations of short-span relationships (Newman, 1966). A quick observation, when verbalized by the nurse, can provide an opening for the patient to express personal concerns relevant to the situation.

Is there a way for me to be effective in the emergency department for the patient who does not dialogue with me (does not allow a mutual relationship)?

An assumption of the theory is that there is an interpenetration of the fields of the nurse and the patient. It is important that you are fully present with the patient in unconditional acceptance of where they are in the situation. This will be felt. You may not see any obvious "results" of your presence, but you can trust that this message is communicated while you are no doubt attending to life and death matters. It may be helpful for you to reflect on the pattern of interaction after the fact.

From M. D. Pharris (1-30-06): My sense is that most of our communication in the emergency setting is nonverbal. It is my hope that my patients feel my love, caring, and open attentiveness before I speak the first word. I attend to being well rested so that I can be fully present when I meet my patients. Obviously if someone has an arterial bleed, a nurse is going to concentrate on stopping the bleeding, which is a technical task—how she or he is present during the process and after is nursing.

Can nurses realistically apply the theory on a day-to-day basis, considering the small amount of time available? I find myself listening to what a patient is saying about what is meaningful and I see the pattern emerge and can gently reflect back.

It sounds like you are applying the theory. The taping and writing down the pattern was initiated as part of the research/learning process. Once you understand it and know what you're doing, it is not necessary. It doesn't take any longer (perhaps less) than other forms of relating to the patient. It's simply a different perspective.

Another nurse responds: I work in a large ICU and used HEC in my practice recently with a young dying man and his wife. I was as transformed as she was. I am so in awe of how application of [the HEC] theory changed my whole perspective and provided the patient's wife with a sense of order in a period of extreme disorder. Words cannot describe the impact this has made on the deceased man's wife, children, family and their community. Nor can any words be found to describe how deeply the experience has touched me.

What would be your intervention with a patient who is suffering from pain?

One would need to interact with the patient in the process of total pattern recognition before it would be evident what action is most appropriate. In HEC, one does not respond to a singular problem without an overall recognition of the client's pattern. Pharris shared an incident when staff in the emergency department referred to her a man who had repeatedly come in for chest pain, which resulted in many electrocardiograms, chest x-rays, blood tests, admissions to rule out a heart attack, ultrasounds of his heart, stress tests, an angiogram, and other diagnostic tests and interventions, without relief of his chest pain. He kept coming back. This night when he returned once again to the emergency department with chest pain, after initial emergency care, Pharris sat down at his side and simply said, "Your heart seems to be hurting" to which he responded with tears in his eyes that his wife had left him and due to a disability he had he was feeling emotionally and physically stuck. They talked through what this meant to him and how he might get on with his life, including a referral to a public health nurse who could come to his home. There was apparent relief of the pain he had been holding onto, as he did not return to the clinic after this encounter. The nurse was able to respond immediately to the most meaningful event in his life.

How would HEC give guidance to caring for patients who smoke, since there has been overwhelming proof that smoking is hazardous to your health?

You can let go of the need to judge the smoking habit as "bad," and simply relate to the patients wherever they are at the time of your encounter. The theory does not assign causality (blame?). It deals with the present and evolving pattern. There are cases where disease occurs in spite of the patient's effort to follow prescribed activities, and contrarily does not occur even in the midst of what medical science considers "bad" habits. From the standpoint of HEC, the nurse is free to be fully present with the patient in whatever situation they encounter.

How does HEC envision caring as linked to evidence-based practice?

The idea of evidence-based practice has been broadened to include not only medical interventions backed by randomized clinical trials, but also diverse forms of evidence, such as qualitative studies of caring and practitioner expertise. Some practicing within the context of HEC might utilize a technique developed in the scientific mode, but the overall practice perspective goes way beyond that kind of "evidence."

Does your concept of energy as non-energetic include absolute consciousness as love?

I have moved away from speaking of energy because it is usually thought of as physical energy, which is related to the material aspects of this world, and I'm talking about a phenomenon that transcends the physical dimensions. Perhaps it is a larger energy that encompasses the whole, and in my way of thinking, that is the informational pattern of consciousness.

Older adulthood seems to be a time of simplification. Is this concept consistent with HEC?

My first response to this question was to contrast the slowing down of physiological aging with the increasing complexity of health as expanding consciousness with age. It has been pointed out to me that I didn't really answer the question, and I have become aware of a deeper meaning of simplification. There is simplicity in the solution to a complex situation. I can attest to the need for simplification in my own life (which I do not consider simple). I am reminded of another example shared with me by a nurse with deep intuitive ability. Her experience with persons with dementia, sometimes associated with older adulthood, was that they have moved to another level of consciousness (beyond our field of comprehension). They occasionally come back and communicate on our level, but for the most part they have transcended our level. I see that as consistent with expanding consciousness.

Do you have thoughts about adapting your methodology to a nonverbal mode?

The HEC method definitely can be adapted to a nonverbal mode. Picard (2000) has utilized creative movement as a way of expressing pattern, and Ruka (2005) has spoken to nonverbal observations of persons with dementia as a way of identifying pattern. Other HEC researcher-practitioners have confidence in their nonverbal communication of caring with evidence that it makes a difference.

What is meant by your concept of pattern?

Pattern is revealed in the client's story of relationships with others and in her or his physiological interactions within and with the environment. It is ongoing and evolving. The relationships depict a recognizable patterning. I'll repeat here a summary of what a number of HEC scholars have to say about participation in the evolving patterning:

Patterning is a process of recognizing and creating meaning in life. It is enduring and evolving. It is a reflection of one's relationships with the significant people in one's life and how those relationships change over time. There is a kind of order inherent in pattern that makes it recognizable but in some sense ineffable. In engaging in the evolving process with clients, we are integral to the process and cannot step outside the process. When we do take the step of describing the evolving pattern in words and diagram, the pattern may appear fixed even though we know it is a living, evolving phenomenon. The words and diagram become metaphors for the pattern—our limited way of conveying the dynamic process. The labeling of pattern with words may mask the specificity of the pattern (as happens in stereotyping). We need to attend to the exactness of the shapes and connections of the relatedness. The dialogue between the nurse and client is a meaning-making, transforming process. [Excerpted from an online dialogue of HEC scholars]

How would you apply your theory to a client diagnosed with cancer? What do you mean by the pattern of the whole?

For the person with cancer (or any other pathology), the question is not so much how it relates to health (in the old sense of the word) but how it is a manifestation of the pattern of the whole. The reason we begin by asking clients to describe what is most meaningful to them is that meaning reveals pattern, and as the client begins to get insight in terms of their pattern, they transcend the old limitations. The pattern of the whole is not an amalgamation of things (like personality, physical appearance, etc.); it is the underlying unseen pattern that manifests itself in observable ways of relating.

How does HEC guide care of a terminal patient?

In being fully present with the patient, the nurse helps the patient experience the meaningfulness of the situation and may help the patient fully experience the transition that death represents. Barron (2005) reported seeing terminal patients thriving in her HEC practice.

Would I be grasping your theory in saying that every encounter is an opportunity to grow as a practitioner and as a person while at the same time helping the client move forward (despite what we know scientifically to be in their best interest)?

Every encounter is an opportunity to grow and for the client to reconsider the trajectory of her or his life. I would not make the assumption that we know what is best for the client, science or no science. The assumption is that the path they choose is integral to expanding consciousness.

How do nurses recognize their own patterns?

The theory does not focus on nurses' looking at their own patterns in isolation. I may have written about getting in touch with one's own pattern but that was meant in relation to the interpenetration of the patterns of the nurse and the patient. I think one needs an interactive participant in order to see the pattern (e.g., the contrast). It may be that a teacher or colleague could provide that facilitative interaction for a student or nurse to learn about oneself, but it would also occur in the encounter with the patient.

What is it about nurses that make them capable of facilitating consciousness expansion in others?

[From Donna, a dialogue participant]: I had a similar question (that is, thinking I'm not qualified to do this), but then I realized our role is not to direct the client's choices, nor to make sense out of his life for him. Using Newman's theory-as-praxis system, our job is to enter into partnership with the client and engage in meaningful dialogue with him as his pattern unfolds. The client guides the discussion, not us. Clarity reveals itself as we project back to the client what we're hearing him say. They determine what's important. . . . the authentic presence of a caring other can facilitate clients' health experience. . . . Nurses frequently encounter clients in moments of disruption and chaos, and we can be privileged to bear witness to their transformation and evolution to a higher level of organization.

[From M. D. Pharris]: I see the nurse-patient relationship as a pure reflection pool through which both the nurse and the patient can see themselves more clearly. In HEC we are clearing ourselves of an intent to "change" or "fix" the other, whether it be patient, family, or community. Rather, we attend to a dialogue where insights into pattern can arise. The wisdom lies within the patient/family/community—it is in the context of the nurse's caring presence that clarity or potential action comes. For traumatized people this is even more essential, because trauma by its very nature, creates a distorted self-image. It is like a circus mirror image where negatives seem very large and positives seem very small. The HEC nurse-patient relationship moves through that distorted image to a clear view of the underlying pattern.

Bibliography

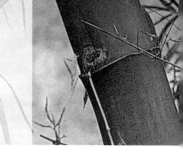

Abbott, E. A. (1952). *Flatland.* New York: Dover.

Albom, M. (1997). *Tuesdays with Morrie.* New York: Doubleday.

American Nurse, The. (September–October, 1998). The official publication of the American Nurses Association.

Arguelles, J. (1984). *Earth ascending, an illustrated treatise on the law governing whole systems.* Santa Fe, NM: Bear & Co.

Arguelles, J. (1987). *The Mayan factor: Path beyond technology.* Santa Fe, NM: Bear & Co.

Arguelles, J. (2002). *Time and the technosphere.* Rochester, VT: Bear and Co.

Arguelles, J., & Arguelles, M. (1985). *Mandala.* Boston: Shambhala.

Bache, C. M. (Undated). What is transformative learning? *Newsletter from Institute of Noetic Sciences,* 2–6.

Bache, C. M. (2000). *Dark night, early dawn.* Albany: State University of New York Press.

Bahnson, C. B., & Bahnson, M. B. (1966). Role of the ego defenses: Denial and repression in the etiology of malignant neoplasm. *Annals of the New York Academy of Science, 125*(3), 827–845.

Barron, A. M. (2001). Entry on listserv, "Dialogue among scholars of the theory of health as expanding consciousness," February 3, 2001.

Barron, A. M. (2005). Suffering, growth, and possibility: Health as expanding consciousness in end-of-life care. In C. Picard & D. Jones (Eds.), *Giving voice to what we know: Margaret Newman's theory of health as expanding consciousness in nursing practice, research, and education.* Sudbury, MA: Jones and Bartlett.

Bateson, G. (1972). *Steps to an ecology of mind.* New York: Ballantine.

Bateson, G. (1979). *Mind and nature.* New York: Bantam Books.

Bentov, I. (1977). *Stalking the wild pendulum.* New York: Dutton.

Bentov, I. (1978). *The mechanics of consciousness.* Paper presented at symposium on New Dimensions of Consciousness, sponsored by Sufi Order in the West, New York, November 17–20.

Bernick, L. (2000). Caring for older adults: Practice guided by Watson's caring-healing model. *Nursing Science Quarterly, 17*(2), 128–134.

Berry, D. (November, 2000). Dialogue, Boston MA.

Berry, D. (2004). An emerging model of behavior change in women maintaining weight loss. *Nursing Science Quarterly, 17*(3), 242–252.

Bohm, D. (1980). *Wholeness and the implicate order.* London: Routledge & Kegan Paul.

Bohm, D. (1992). On dialogue. *IONS Noetic Sciences Review,* No. 23, 16–18.

Bohm, D. (1992). *Thought as a system.* London: Routledge.

Bortoft, H. (1986). *Goethe's scientific consciousness.* Kent, England: Institute for Cultural Research (Monograph Series No. 22).

Bortoft, H. (1996). *The wholeness of nature: Goethe's way toward a science of conscious participation in nature.* New York: Lindisfarne.

Brain/Mind Bulletin, 1986. (Prigogine)

Briggs, J., & Peat, F. D. (1990). *Turbulent mirror.* New York: Harper & Row.

Bronson, M. C. (2006). Getting real: The praxis of integral education. *Re-Vision, 28*(3), 2–3.

Butrin, J. (1992). Cultural diversity in the nurse-client encounter. *Clinical Nursing Research, 1*(3), 238–251.

Capasso, V. A. (2005). The theory is the practice: An exemplar. In C. Picard & D. Jones (Eds.), *Giving voice to what we know: Margaret Newman's theory of health as expanding consciousness in nursing practice, research, and education* (pp. 65–72). Sudbury MA: Jones and Bartlett.

Capra, F. (1982). *The turning point: Science, society, and the rising culture.* New York: Simon & Schuster.

Chase, S. K. (2001). Response to "The concept of nursing presence: State of the science." *Scholarly Inquiry for Nursing Practice: An International Journal, 15*(4), 323–327.

Cooper, A.,& Elgin, D. (2002-2003) Peril and promise. *IONS Noetic Sciences Review,* No. 62, 8–15+.

De Quincey, C. (1998). *Intersubjectivity: Exploring consciousness from the second-person perspective.* Unpublished manuscript.

De Quincey, C. (2005). *Radical knowing: Understanding consciousness through relationship.* Rochester, VT: Park Street Press.

Donaldson, S. K., & Crowley, D. M. (1978). The discipline of nursing. *Nursing Outlook, 26*(2), 113–120.

Donoso, S. (2003). The power of presence: An interview with spiritual teacher Eckhart Tolle. *IONS Noetic Sciences Review,* No. 63 (March-May), 14–17.

Doona, M. E., Chase, S. K., & Haggerty, L. A. (1999). Nursing presence: As real as a Milky Way bar. *Journal of Holistic Nursing, 17*(1), 54–70.

Edwards, M. G. (2002). "The way up is the way down": Integral sociocultural studies and cultural evolution. *ReVision, 28*(2) Winter 2002.

Elgin, D. (2002–2003). On simplicity and humanity's future: Peril and promise. *IONS Noetic Sciences Review,* No. 62, 8–15.

Elias, D. (1997). It's time to change our minds: An introduction to transformative learning. *ReVision, 20*(1), 2–6.

Emerson, R. W. (1860, rev. 1876). Beauty. In *Nature,* published as part of *Nature; Addresses and Lectures.* Accessed January 12, 2007 from http://www.emersoncentral.com/beauty.htm 01/12/2007.

Endo, E. (1998). Pattern recognition as a nursing intervention with Japanese women with ovarian cancer. *Advances in Nursing Science, 20*(4), 49–61.

Endo, E. (2004). Nursing praxis within Margaret Newman's theory of health as expanding consciousness. *Nursing Science Quarterly, 17*(2), 110–115.

Endo, E. (2006). Personal communication.

Endo, E., Minegishi, H., Kubo, S. (2005). Creating action research teams: a praxis model of care. In C. Picard & D. Jones (Eds.), *Giving voice to what we know: Margaret Newman's theory of health as expanding consciousness in nursing practice, research, and education* (pp. 143–151). Sudbury, MA: Jones and Bartlett.

Endo, E, Miyahara, T., Suzuki, S., Ohmasa, T. (2005). Caring partnering between nurse educator and practicing nurses. *Nursing Science Quarterly, 18*(3), 138–145.

Endo, E., Nitta, N., Inayoshi, M., Saito, R., Takemura, K., Minegishi, H., Kubo, S., & Kondon, M. (2000). Pattern recognition as a caring partnership in families with cancer. *Journal of Advanced Nursing, 32*(3), 603–610.

Endo, E., Takaki, M., Abe, K., Terashima, K., & Nitta, N. (2007). *Creating a helping model with nursing students who want to quit smoking: Patterning in a nursing student-teacher partnership based on M. Newman's theory of health.* Paper presented at The Power of Caring : The Gateway to Healing, 29th annual International Association for Human Caring Conference, St. Louis, MO, May 16–19, 2007.

Falkenstern, S. (2003). *Nursing facilitation of health as expanding consciousness in families who have a child with special health care needs.*

Unpublished PhD dissertation. The Pennsylvania State University, University Park, PA.

Fawcett. J. (1993). *Analysis and evaluation of nursing theories.* Philadelphia: F. A. Davis.

Ferguson, M. (1980). *The aquarian conspiracy: Personal and social transformation in the 1980s.* Los Angeles: J. P. Tarcher.

Ferguson, M. (1983). Brain/Mind Bulletin.

Flanagan, J. (November 2000). Dialogue. Boston MA.

Flanagan, J. (2005). Creating a healing environment for staff and patients in a pre-surgery clinic. In C. Picard & D. Jones (Eds.), *Giving voice to what we know: Margaret Newman's theory of health as expanding consciousness in nursing practice, research, and education.* Sudbury, MA: Jones and Bartlett.

Fox, M. (1988). *The coming of the cosmic Christ.* San Francisco: Harper.

Friedman, N. (1990, 1994). *Bridging science and spirit.* St. Louis: Living Lake Books.

Friedman, T. L. (2005). *The world is flat: A brief history of the 21st century.* New York: Farrar, Straus & Giroux.

Fuller, R. B. (1975). *Synergetics.* New York: Macmillan.

Geschwind, N., & Galaburda, A. M. (1985). Cerebral lateralization - Biological mechanisms, associations, and pathology: III. A hypothesis and a program for research. *Archives of Neurology, 42*(July), 634–654.

Gilbert, R. J. (2006). Sacred geometry. *Shift: At the Frontiers of Consciousness.* No. 11, June–August, 15–19.

Goodman, J. (1979). *We are the earthquake generation.* New York: Berkley.

Goodwin, B. (1991). The generative order of life. *IONS Noetic Sciences Review,* No. 18, Spring–Summer, 14–20.

Grand, I. J. (2005). The practice of embodied emergence: Integral education in a counseling psychology program. *ReVision, 28*(2), 35–42.

Grossinger, R. (2004). Healing as art and technology. *Shift: At the Frontiers of Consciousness.* June–August, 10–15.

Grossman, N. (2002), Who's afraid of life after death? *IONS Noetic Sciences Review, 61,* 30–35.

Harman, W. W. (1988). The persistent puzzle: The need for a basic restructuring of science. *IONS Noetic Science Review,* No. 8, 22–25.

Harman, W. W. (1988). The transpersonal challenge to the scientific paradigm: The need for a restructuring of science. *ReVision, 11*(2), 13–21.

Harman, W. W. (1993). How do we know what we think we know? Toward an epistemology of consciousness, *IONS Noetic Sciences Review, 27,* 72–76.

Harman, W. W. (1993). Toward an adequate science of consciousness. *IONS Noetic Sciences Review, 27,* 77–78.

Havel, V. (1983). *Letters to Olga.* New York: Henry Holt.

Hiley, B. J. (2002). On quantum mechanics and the implicate order. Interview conducted by M. Perus. (http://goertzel.org/dynaphapsyc/1997/interview.html).

Johnson, D. E. (1961). The significance of nursing care. *The American Journal of Nursing, 61*(11), 63–66.

Jones, Dorothy. (2006) Personal communication.

Jonsdottir, H. (1998). Life patterns of people with chronic obstructive pulmonary disease: Isolation and being closed in. *Nursing Science Quarterly, 11*(4), 160–166.

Jonsdottir, H., Litchfield, M., & Pharris, M. D. (2003). Partnership in practice. *Research and Theory for Nursing Practice: An International Journal, 17*(1), 51–63.

Khan, P. V. I. (1978). *Holistic meditation.* New Dimensions of Consciousness, held in New York City, November 17–20, 1978.

Kidd, S. M. (1996). *The dance of the dissident daughter: A woman's journey from Christian tradition to the sacred feminine.* San Francisco: Harper.

Kiser-Larson, N. (2002). Life pattern of Native women experiencing breast cancer. *International Journal for Human Caring, 6*(2), 61–68.

Kohanov, L. (2003). *Riding between the worlds: Expanding our potential through the way of the horse.* Novato, CA: New World Library.

Kremer, J. W. (1992). The dark night of the scholar: Reflections on culture and ways of knowing. *ReVision, 14*(4), 169–178.

Kremer, J. W. (1997). Transforming learning transforming. *ReVision, 20*(1), 7–14.

Kunz, D. vG. (1991). *The personal aura.* Wheaton, IL: Quest.

Lamendola, F. (1998). *Patterns of the caregiving experiences of selected nurses in hospice and HIV/AIDS care.* PhD Dissertation, University of Minnesota, Minneapolis.

Lamendola, F., & Newman, M. A. (1994). The paradox of HIV/AIDS as expanding consciousness. *Advances in Nursing Science, 16*(3), 13–21.

Lather, P. (1986). Research as praxis. *Harvard Educational Review, 56*(3), 257–277.

LeShan, L. (1989). Cancer as a turning point. *IONS Noetic Sciences Review, 11*, 22–28.

Lindbergh, C. (1972). Man's potential. In C. Muses & A. M. Young (Eds.), *Consciousness and reality: The human pivot point*. New York: Outerbridge & Lazard.

Litchfield, M. (1999). Practice wisdom. *Advances in Nursing Science, 22*(2), 62–73.

Litchfield, M. (2004). *Achieving health in a rural community: A case study of nurse-community partnership*. Wellington, New Zealand: Litchfield Healthcare Associates.

Melnechenko, K. L. (2003). To make a difference: Nursing presence. *Nursing Forum, 38*(2), 18–24.

Miles, R. B. (1998). Our evolving views of health and illness: What does it all mean? *Connections*, No. 3(February), Institute of Noetic Sciences, 7–9.

Miller, M.A., & Douglas, M. R. (1998). Presencing: Nurses commitment to caring for dying persons. *International Journal for Human Caring, 2*(3), 24–31.

Mishel, M. H. (1990). Reconceptualization of the uncertainty in illness theory. *Image, 22*(4), 256–261.

Moch, S. D. (1990). Health within the experience of breast cancer. *Journal of Advanced Nursing, 15*, 1426–1435.

Montuori, H. (2006). The quest for a new education: From oppositional identities to creative inquiry. *ReVision, 28*(3), 4-20.

Moss, R. (1981). *The I that is we*. Millbrae, CA: Celestial Arts.

Muses, C. (1972). The exploration of consciousness. In Muses, C. & Young, A. M. (Eds.), *Consciousness and reality: The human pivot point*. New York: Outerbridge & Lazard.

Muses, C. (1978). Paper presented at symposium on New Dimensions of Consciousness, Sufi Order in the West, New York City, November 17–20.

Muses, C. (1985). *Destiny and control in human systems*. Boston-Dordrecht-Lancaster: Kluwer-Nifhoff.

Muses, C., & Young, A. M. (Eds.). (1972). *Consciousness and reality: The human pivot point*. New York: Outerbridge and Lazard.

Musker, K. M. (2005). *Life patterns of women transitioning through menopause*. PhD dissertation, Loyola University, Chicago.

Neill, J. (2002a). Transcendence and transformation in the life patterns of women living with rheumatoid arthritis. *Advances in Nursing Science, 24*(4), 27–47.

Neill, J. (2002b). From practice to caring praxis through Newman's theory of health as expanding consciousness: A personal journey. *International Journal for Human Caring, 6*, 48–54.

Newman, M. A. (1966). Identifying and meeting patients' needs in short-span nurse-patient relationships. *Nursing Forum, 5*(1), 76–86.

Newman, M. A. (1972). Time estimation in relation to gait tempo. *Perceptual and Motor Skills, 34*, 359–366.

Newman, M. A. (1978). *Toward a theory of health.* Paper presented at Nurse Educator Conference, New York, NY.

Newman, M. A. (1979). *Theory development in nursing.* Philadelphia: F. A. Davis.

Newman, M. A. (1982). Time as an index of consciousness with age. *Nursing Research, 31*, 290–293.

Newman, M. A. (1983). Nursing diagnosis: Looking at the whole. *American Journal of Nursing, 84*, 1496–1499.

Newman, M. A. (1986). *Health as expanding consciousness.* St. Louis: Mosby.

Newman, M. A. (1987). Aging as increasing complexity. *Journal of Gerontological Nursing, 13*(9), 16–18.

Newman, M. A.(1990). Newman's theory of health as praxis. *Nursing Science Quarterly, 3*(1), 37–41.

Newman, M. A. (1994). *Health as expanding consciousness* (2nd ed.). Sudbury, MA: Jones and Bartlett (NLN Press).

Newman, M. A. (1995a). Recognizing a pattern of expanding consciousness in persons with cancer. In M. A. Newman, *A developing discipline: Selected works of Margaret Newman* (pp. 159–171). Sudbury, MA: Jones and Bartlett (NLN Press).

Newman, M. A. (1995b). *A developing discipline: Selected works of Margaret Newman.* Sudbury, MA: Jones and Bartlett (NLN Press).

Newman, M. A. (1997). Evolution of the theory of health as expanding consciousness. *Nursing Science Quarterly, 10*(1), 22–25.

Newman, M. A. (1997). Experiencing the whole. *Advances in Nursing Science, 20*(1), 34–39.

Newman, M. A. (2002a). Caring in the human health experience. *International Journal for Human Caring, 6*(2), 8–12.

Newman, M. A. (2002b). The pattern that connects. *Advances in Nursing Science, 24*(3), 1–7.

Newman, M. A. (2003). A world of no boundaries. *Advances in Nursing Science, 26*(4), 240–245.

Newman, M. A., & Gaudiano, J. K. (1984). Depression as an explanation for decreased subjective time in the elderly. *Nursing Research, 33,* 137–139.

Newman, M. A., Lamb, G. S., & Michaels, C. (1991). Nurse case management: The coming together of theory and practice. *Nursing & Health Care, 12*(8), 404–408.

Newman, M. A., & Moch, S. D. (1991). Life patterns of persons with coronary heart disease. *Nursing Science Quarterly, 4,* 161–167.

Newman, M. A., Sime, A. M., & Corcoran-Perry, S. A. (1991). The focus of the discipline of nursing. *Advances in Nursing Science, 14*(1), 1–6.

Nichols, M. (2004). AARP Magazine, January & February, p. 40.

Nightingale, F. (1859). *Notes on nursing.* Facsimile of first edition by J. B. Lippincott Co.

Noveletsky-Rosenthal, H. (1996). *Pattern recognition in older adults living with chronic illness.* PhD dissertation, Boston College, Chestnut Hill, MA.

Parker, M. (2001). *Nursing theories and nursing practice.* Philadelphia: F. A. Davis.

Parse, R. R. (1987). *Nursing science: Major paradigms, theories and critiques.* Philadelphia: Saunders.

Parse, R. R. (1998). *The human becoming school of thought.* Thousand Oaks, CA: Sage.

Paul, M. I., Akers, A., Dunn, D., & Brodsky, A. B. (1986). Music, language, and "uncertainty receptors," *IS Journal #2,* 3–10.

Peat, F. D. (1991). *The philosopher's stone: Chaos synchronicity, and the hidden order of the world.* New York: Bantam Books.

Pharris, M. D. (2002). Coming to know ourselves as community through a nursing partnership with adolescents convicted of murder. *Advances in Nursing Science, 24*(3), 21–42.

Pharris, M. D. (2005). Engaging with communities in a pattern recognition process. In C. Picard & D. Jones (Eds.), *Giving voice to what we know: Margaret Newman's theory of health as expanding consciousness in nursing practice, research, and education.* Sudbury, MA: Jones and Bartlett.

Pharris, M. D. (Undated). *A community-based action research collaboration between the College of St. Catherine and the National Community Center of Excellence in Women's Health/NorthPoint Health & Wellness Center.* Minneapolis, MN.

Phillips, J. (1990) The different views of health. *Nursing Science Quarterly,* *3*(3), 103–104.

Picard, C. (2000). Pattern of expanding consciousness in mid-life women: Creative movement and the narrative as modes of expression. *Nursing Science Quarterly, 13*(2), 150–158.

Picard, C., & Jones, D. (2005). *Giving voice to what we know: Margaret Newman's theory of health as expanding consciousness in nursing practice, research, and education.* Sudbury MA: Jones and Bartlett.

Picard, C., & Mariolis, T. (2005). Praxis as a mirroring process: Teaching psychiatric nursing grounded in Newman's health as expanding consciousness. In C. Picard & D. Jones (Eds.), *Giving voice to what we know: Margaret Newman's theory of health as expanding consciousness in nursing practice, research, and education.* Sudbury, MA: Jones and Bartlett.

Prigogine, I. (1976). Order through fluctuation: Self-organization and social system. In E. Jantsch & C. H. Waddington (Eds.), *Evolution and consciousness* (pp. 93–133). Reading, MA: Addison-Wesley.

Prigogine, I. (1986). *Brain/mind bulleting* (p. 2), September 8, 1986.

Prigogine, I., & Stengers, I. (1984). *Order out of chaos: Man's new dialogue with nature.* Shambhala.

Reed, P. G. (1991). Toward a nursing theory of self-transcendence: Deductive reformation using developmental theories. *Advances in Nursing Science, 13*(4), 64–77.

Reinharz, S. (1983). Phenomenology as a dynamic process. *Phenomenology and Pedagogy, 1*(1), 77–79

Rogers, M. (1970). *An introduction to the theoretical basis of nursing.* Philadelphia: F. A. Davis.

Rogers, M. (1995). *Her own eulogy.* Audiotape recording (in conversation with Marcia Anderson).

Rosa, K. C. (2006). A process model of healing and personal transformation in persons with chronic skin wounds. *Nursing Science Quarterly, 19*(4), 349–358.

Roy, C. (2007). Knowledge as universal cosmic imperative. In C. Roy & D. Jones (Eds.), *Nursing knowledge development and clinical practice* (pp. 145–161). New York: Springer.

Roy, C. & Jones, D. (Eds.). (2007). *Nursing knowledge development and clinical practice.* New York: Springer.

Ruka, S. (2005). Creating balance: Rhythms and patterns in people with dementia living in a nursing home. In C. Picard & D. Jones (Eds.),

Giving voice to what we know: Margaret Newman's theory of health as expanding consciousness in nursing practice, research, and education. Sudbury, MA: Jones and Bartlett.

Russell, P. (1992). *The white hole in time: Our future evolution and the meaning of now.* San Francisco: HarperCollins.

Sakalys, J. A. (2003). Restoring the patient's voice: The therapeutics of illness narrative. *Journal of Holistic Nursing, 21*(3), 228–241.

Schlitz, M. (2004). Seeding a new model of medicine. *Shift: At the Frontiers of Consciousness,* June–August, 8–9.

Schlitz, M., Taylor, E., & Lewis, N. (1998) Toward a noetic model of medicine. *IONS Noetic Sciences Review,* No. 47, 44–52.

Schwartz, S. A. (2006). Opening to the infinite. *Shift: At the Frontiers of Consciousness,* No. 10, 28–31.

Sheilds, L. E., & Lindsey, A. E. (1998). Community health promotion nursing practice. *Advances in Nursing Science, 20*(4), 23–36.

Sheldrake, R. (1983). *A new science of life.* Los Angeles: Tarcher.

Shostak, D., & Whitehouse, P. J. (1999). Diseases of meaning, manifestations of health, and metaphor. *The Journal of Alternative and Complementary Medicine, 5*(6), 495–502.

Silva, M., Sorrell, J., & Sorrell C. (1995). From Carper's pattern of knowing to ways of being. An ontological philosophical shift in nursing. *Advances in Nursing Science, 18*(1), 1–13.

Skolimowski, H. (1994). *The participatory mind: A new theory of knowledge and of the universe(* Arkana). Penguin Books.

Smith, K. (2006). Bioenergetics: A new science of healing. *Shift: At the Frontiers of Consciousness,* No. 10, 11–13.

Smith, M. (1999). Caring and the science of unitary human beings. *Advances in Nursing Science, 21*(4), 14–28.

Smith, T. D. (2001). The concept of nursing presence: State of the science. *Scholarly Inquiry for Nursing Practice: An International Journal, 15*(4), 299–322.

Spradlin, W. W., & Porterfield, P. (1984). *The search for certainty.* New York: Springer-Verlag.

Stone, H. (1978). *Holism: A new vision of man, a new vision of health.* Paper presented at Conference on Holistic Perspectives: A Renaissance in Medicine and Health Care, Philadelphia, November 12.

Tang, Y. (1997). Fostering transformation through differences: The synergic inquiry (SI) framework. *ReVision, 20*(1), 15–19.

Tarnas, R. (1998). The great initiation. *IONS Noetic Sciences Review,* No. 47, 24–31+.

Tarnas, R. (2002). Is the modern psyche undergoing a rite of passage? *ReVision, 24*(3), 2–10.

Taylor, A. (1972). Meaning and matter. In C. Muses & A. M. Young (Eds.), *Consciousness and reality: The human pivot point.* New York: Outerbridge & Lazard.

Taylor, D. (2001). *Tell me a story: The life-shaping power of our stories.* St. Paul, MN: Bog Walk Press.

Thompson, W. I., (Ed.). (1991). *Gaia 2 emergence, The new science of becoming.* Lindisfarne.

Tomey, A., & Alligood, M. (1998). *Nurse theorists and their work.* St. Louis: Mosby.

Tommet, P. (2003). Nurse-parent dialogue: Illuminating the evolving pattern of families with children who are medically fragile. *Nursing Science Quarterly, 16*(3), 239–246.

Watson, J. (1988). *Nursing: Human science and human care—A theory of nursing.* New York: National League for Nursing.

Watson, J. (1999). *Postmodern nursing and beyond.* Edinburgh: Churchill Livingstone.

Watson-Gegeo, K. A. (2005). Teaching to transform and the dark side of "being professional." *ReVision, 28*(2), 43–48.

Weber, R. (1984). Compassion, rootedness and detachment: Their role in healing. A conversation with Dora Kunz. *ReVision, 7*(1), 76–82.

Whitmont, E. C. (1994). Form and information. *IONS Noetic Sciences Review,* No. 31, 11–18.

Wilber, K. (1979). *No boundary: Eastern and western approaches to personal growth.* Boulder, CO: Shambhala.

Wilber, K. (1998). *The marriage of sense and soul: Integrating science and religion.* New York: Random House.

Wilber, K. (2000). *Sex, ecology, spirituality: The spirit of evolution.* Shambhala.

Young, A. (1976). *The reflexive universe: Evolution of consciousness.* San Francisco: Briggs.

INDEX